A Step-by-Step Guide to Clinical Trials

Marilyn Mulay
R.N., M.S., OCN®
University of California at Los Angeles

JONES AND BARTLETT PUBLISHERS
Sudbury, Massachusetts
BOSTON   TORONTO   LONDON   SINGAPORE

World Headquarters
Jones and Bartlett Publishers
40 Tall Pine Drive
Sudbury, MA 01776
978-443-5000
info@jbpub.com
www.jbpub.com

Jones and Bartlett Publishers Canada
2406 Nikanna Road
Mississauga, ON L5C 2W6
CANADA

Jones and Bartlett Publishers International
Barb House, Barb Mews
London W6 7PA
UK

PRODUCTION CREDITS
ACQUISITIONS EDITOR: John Danielowich
PRODUCTION EDITOR: Linda S. DeBruyn
EDITORIAL/PRODUCTION ASSISTANT: Christine Tridente
V.P., MANUFACTURING AND INVENTORY: Therese Bräuer
TYPESETTING: Modern Graphics, Inc.
TEXT DESIGN: Modern Graphics, Inc.
COVER DESIGN: Stephanie Torta
PRINTING AND BINDING: Malloy Lithographing

Library of Congress Cataloging-in-Publication Data
Mulay, Marilyn.
   A step-by-step guide to clinical trials / Marilyn Mulay.
      p. cm.
   Includes bibliographical references and index.
   ISBN 0-7637-1569-7
   1. Clinical trials. I. Title.
R853.C55 M84 2000
619—dc21   00-062680

Printed in the United States of America
10 09 08 07 06   10 9 8 7 6 5 4 3 2

The selection and dosage of drugs presented in this book are in accord with standards accepted at the time of publication. The authors, editors, and publisher have made every effort to provide accurate information. However, research, clinical practice, and government regulations often change the accepted standard in this field. Before administering any drug, the reader is advised to check the manufacturer's product information sheet for the most up-to-date recommendations on dosage, precautions, and contraindications. This is especially important in the case of drugs that are new or seldom used.

To all of the brave patients
who volunteer for clinical trials.
Without your courage and participation,
the search for answers would be futile.

Contents

PAR**T II**   *Setting the Foundation*

PAR**T III**   *The Clinical Side*

Preface

The greatest thing in this world is not so much where we are,
but in what direction we are moving.
—Oliver Wendell Holmes

Clinical research is the foundation to find the answers to many of the diseases that confront the world's population. The information gathered in clinical trials is important to the development of useful treatments for a variety of devastating illnesses. The goal is not only to lengthen life expectancy but also to improve the quality of that life. Clinicians are often frustrated when the scope of their knowledge stops short of saving a patient's life. In response to those frustrations, research is being conducted at a furious pace in academic medical centers and biotechnological companies worldwide.

Pharmaceutical companies have been growing, merging, expanding, and searching for talented scientists to open the doors to the mystery of disease and its control. Once scientists identify and test new compounds in the laboratory, the drugs need to be tested in human trials. All drugs or treatments must be subjected to the rigors of objective testing before any claim can be made to substantive benefit. The importance of designing and conducting safe clinical trials in the development of drugs or medical devices cannot be overstated. Yet, the lack of formal and consistent training in this area is painfully evident. Although the U.S. Food and Drug Administration has issued guidelines for clinical testing, the interpretation and implementation of the guidelines varies widely. Indeed, the procedures used to conduct clinical research vary from one organization to the next.

At many research centers, the experience of the principal investigator, the study coordinator, or the representative of the pharmaceutical company who has designed the trial often dictates the procedures. The result can be biased, confusing, or—worse—unevaluable data. A potentially useful drug or device should not be denied to the public because of the lack of training or knowledge of those conducting the research. At the same time, the public must be protected from unscrupulous or unreliable research, whether it is done knowingly or unwittingly.

Clinical research is a logical process. There is nothing mysterious or really difficult about it. If done well, a great deal of time and money can be saved, and important treatments can get to the marketplace sooner, giving new treatment options to clinicians and potential benefits to patients.

Establishing an organized system to conduct clinical trials has been a long-standing need. The purpose of this book is to share years of experience and knowledge as well as to advance the cause of clinical research. Since this approach to clinical trials was developed for a phase I program in oncology, the book has been written from that perspective. It has been said that oncology patients in a phase I study present one of the greatest challenges to a research team in terms of patient management as well as defining toxicities. Adaptation of the information presented here for use in other programs and phases of clinical trials should be relatively easy.

Designed as a step-by-step guide, the book walks you through clinical trials from beginning to end. Part I, The Business of Research, discusses the design of clinical trials, and defines components of a protocol, regulatory requirements, and budgeting and contract processes. Part II, Setting the Foundation, builds a clear pathway to a well-organized clinical trial. The Clinical Side, Part III, gives stepping stones for successful patient enrollment and safe patient care, while Part IV, The Data Side, smoothes the road and shortens the distance to collecting and recording *clean* data. Organizational Issues are discussed in Part V to pave the way to a successful research program.

The field of clinical research offers exciting opportunities not only for healthcare professionals but also for people trained in other disciplines. It offers the fulfillment of working with patients who are courageous and appreciative and the challenge and personal satisfaction that come from seeking answers to seemingly unanswerable questions. Knowing that you have made a significant contribution to clinical research and possibly future treatments for serious illnesses is very rewarding.

Clinical research offers hope for today and promise for tomorrow.

Acknowledgments

Many, many thanks to:

the Cancer Therapy Development team at UCLA—Lee Rosen, Joseph Brown, Leny Kadib, Mandy Parson, Laura Reiswig, Andre Mayers, Bernadette Laxa, Natasha Gicanov, Jennifer Mickey, Luis Hernandez, Mae Gordon, and Allison Kaplan. Your support and encouragement not only got this book started but sustained the effort until completion.

those who, in addition to their support, helped to define the content and provided editorial assistance—Cynthia Dunn, Pat and John Soller, and John White: Teresa and the editorial staff of Jones and Bartlett, including John Danielowich and Linda DeBruyn; and the editorial staff at Modern Graphics, particularly Michael Granger.

my family, James and Trisha Rudnick, and Dana and Gus Lira. Special thanks to Dana for her invaluable legal counsel.

And a very special thanks to Don Friedman whose continued encouragement and unrelenting support made this book a reality.

PART I

The Business of Research

- *The Cancer Problem*

- *The Protocol Process*

- *Regulatory Issues*

- *The Budget*

- *The Contract*

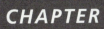

The Cancer Problem

Cancer is a group of distinct diseases with one thing in common. In all of these diseases, cells grow and spread in an uncontrolled manner. The affected cells lose the natural protective mechanisms that would normally limit their growth and cause them to die.

In the United States, cancer is the second leading case of death after heart disease. It is estimated that 1.2 million new cases of cancer will be diagnosed in 2000 and that 552,000 Americans will die because of it. However, there are also approximately 8.4 million Americans alive today who are cancer survivors.[1] Some of these people are considered cured while others are said to be in remission or may still have some evidence of disease.

We know that a variety of factors are implicated in certain cancers: some factors are controllable and others are not. For example, cancers caused by cigarette smoking or alcohol abuse could be prevented by avoiding these behaviors. Tobacco is responsible for at least 30 percent of all cancer deaths, or approximately 430,700 deaths each year.[2] bout 3 percent of all cancer deaths can be attributed to alcohol, and the use of both alcohol and tobacco has a negative, synergistic effect on many cancers.[3] Further, scientific evidence shows that about one-third of cancer deaths are related to nutrition. Diets high in fat have been implicated in breast cancer and high fat, low fiber diets play a role in colorectal cancer.[1] Many of the 1.3 million cases of skin cancer diag-

3

nosed in the United States each year could be prevented with appropriate protection from the sun.[1] Despite these controllable factors, genetic disposition also plays a significant role in cancer, particularly in colorectal and breast cancers.

Why a cancer develops is essentially unknown. The most commonly accepted theory is that cancer develops in several phases. **Initiation** is the first phase. Normally, a cell replicates through a series of complex chemical instructions. In cancer, the DNA is damaged either by genetic mutation or a *carcinogen*. The cell may repair itself or remain permanently changed without consequence of cancer. If the cell becomes transformed and the initiator is a complete carcinogen (that is, if it acts as an initiator and promoter), then a cancer cell line results.

Promotion, the second phase, is a process by which carcinogens are introduced to a cell. If a cell that has already encountered an initiator then comes in contact with a promoter, a succession of events begins that allows the cell to defy its natural life cycle and grow uncontrollably, becoming immortal. If the immune system of the host, or patient, cannot halt the mutated cell, then the cell replicates millions of times, forming a mass. When it achieves a size of at least 1 centimeter, the mass can be detected by either palpation or radiological examination. Such a mass may take years to develop. The official diagnosis of cancer is made after cells from the mass are retrieved and under a microscope, are determined to be cancerous by a pathologist.

If the development of cancer stopped at the promotion phase, most cancers could be removed and would have little more effect than the common cold. Unfortunately, most cancers are not detected before the last phase, **progression**. During this phase, the cancer spreads from its original location, by either **invasion** or **metastasis**, via the lymph or circulatory system.

■ Treatment

Whenever possible, surgery is used to remove a cancer that has not spread and is contained within an accessible area of the body. Often, surgery is followed by radiation and/or chemotherapy to safeguard against **micrometastasis**, or the spread of diseased cells beyond the surgical resection. Such treatment after complete surgical resection and in the absence of known disease is called **adjuvant therapy**.

If disease is not surgically resectable or has already spread to other sites, then **systemic chemotherapy** is the treatment of choice. **Chemotherapy** is the use of a chemical or drug to treat a symptom or illness. It can be as simple as taking two aspirins for a headache. In the context of cancer treatment, however, the word *chemotherapy* connotes such negative images as hair loss, nausea, vomiting, and suppression of the immune system, among others. The goal of cancer chemotherapy is to kill all cells with toxic drugs, with the hope that only normal cells will grow back.

Chemotherapy is given in a variety of ways, most commonly by intravenous infusion. It also can be given orally, intraperitoneally (directly into the abdomen), or intrathecally (into the spinal canal).

Radiation is also used in the treatment of a variety of cancers. It can be used to shrink a mass prior to surgery, to treat an unresectable lesion, for pain control, and/or to treat bony metastases. If the radiation field includes bone containing a lot of bone marrow (for example, the pelvis or sternum), the patient's blood counts can be significantly and negatively affected. Often there is irritation to the skin and sometimes to the structures that underlie the radiated area. A maximum amount of radiation can be given to an area without causing permanent damage to the normal tissues. Once that level has been reached, the area cannot be radiated again.

In the past 40 years, many new chemotherapeutic agents have been developed and used in the treatment of cancer. In solid tumors (not leukemia, multiple myeloma, lymphoma), there have been modest gains in prolonging the life of patients with cancer. However, there has been no significant impact on survival. For the last decade, therefore, cancer researchers have focused on studying what makes the cancer cell different from the normal cell. It is that difference which is the focus of many of the new drugs that are being developed. Because these novel drugs specifically target the unique properties of a cancer cell, they do not appear to be as toxic to the patient as were the earlier drugs. Still, clinical trials and careful data collection are needed to determine the efficacy of these drugs.

■ Clinical Trials

A **clinical trial** is a research method used to test in humans drugs that have shown positive activity in the laboratory and in animal studies. In the United States, the U.S. Food and Drug Administration (FDA) oversees human drug testing to safeguard the public from dangerous compounds and unscrupulous investigators.[4] The thalidomide disaster is an event in recent history that poignantly and sadly defines the devastating consequences of the potential dangers of drug testing. Thalidomide was used in the early 1960s to treat nausea and vomiting during the first trimester of pregnancy. Unfortunately, it also caused devastating birth defects in the children of the women who used it.

Although animal testing seeks to define what toxicities may arise in humans, there is often little correlation. Many promising laboratory results seen in animals cannot be duplicated in human subjects or the side effects of those compounds make their use in humans unacceptable. Therefore, before new drugs can be made available to patients, the FDA mandates that the drugs undergo rigorous clinical trials that are conducted in four phases.

Once a new drug has completed laboratory and animal testing, the drug's developer (sponsor) applies to the FDA for an **IND**, or an investigational new drug, number. The sponsor writes a protocol for the clinical trial with certain objectives in mind. The protocol must scientifically prove the objectives of the study while also providing for patient safety. The sponsor identifies one or more clinical sites, usually academic medical centers, to execute the protocol.

Phase I Study

The objective of a phase I clinical trial is safety. It answers the following questions:

1. What is the correct dose of the drug?
2. What are the side effects?
3. How is the drug metabolized?

Phase I trials are always single-agent studies because combining a new, untested drug with another compound could produce unknown drug-to-drug interactions. It also would be impossible to define which side effects were related to the study drug only and which were related to another drug or to the combination.

There are several ways to determine the safe starting dose in a phase I study. One of the ways uses information from the preclinical work. Typically, the mice are given increasing doses of the drug until the mice die, the lethal dose. The starting dose for humans is then calculated by taking $1/10^{th}$ of the dose that killed 10 percent of the mice. This is called the LD_{10}. The starting dose, and perhaps several dose escalations beyond that, are generally believed to be subtherapeutic, that is not high enough to elicit a response. However, responses have been seen at doses lower than the therapeutic dose in the animals and the safety of the human subjects is paramount.

In a typical phase I design, three patients are enrolled at one dose level and observed for a full cycle, usually 3 to 4 weeks. If no serious toxicities are noted, the dose is then escalated and three more patients are enrolled at the higher dose.

The percentage of dose escalation can vary from 33 percent to 100 percent. A protocol defines the percent of escalation based on the toxicities seen in the preceding cohort (group of patients). When a toxicity or side effect occurs in a particular patient, the principal investigator must determine whether its causality is likely to be related to the study drug or rather from the underlying disease. If the drug is not implicated then the dose will be escalated, perhaps by as much as 100 percent. However, if there has been a **grade 2** (moderate) **toxicity** that is possibly related to the study drug, then the dose will be escalated only by 30 to 40 percent.

Once the principal investigator and the sponsor determine the new dose level, three more patients are enrolled, and the group is observed for another 3- to 4-week cycle. As before, if no serious toxicities occur, the dose is again escalated and three more patients are enrolled. The process continues until a **dose-limiting toxicity** (DLT), which might be as benign as a severe headache or as serious as death, occurs. It is expected that before something as devastating as death occurs, some warning signs will be seen, but this may not always be the case.

For most toxicities, once the drug is withdrawn, the **serious adverse event** (SAE) stops, generally without sequelae. When the DLT is found, the dose is reduced to the preceding dose level, and the **maximum-tolerated dose** (MTD) is declared. At this time, six more patients are typically enrolled at the MTD to ensure that the MTD dose is safe and then if no new toxicities are observed at that dose, the study is closed to further enrollment. Patients who are in the study continue to receive the drug as long as their disease does not progress.

Pharmacokinetic (PK) blood samples are usually drawn during phase I and sometimes during phase II studies. Pharmacokinetic sampling seeks to identify the drug's **metabolites** and its **half-life**, or the time required for the body to eliminate half of the drug.

In order to understand how a drug works in humans, analysis of the drug's metabolites is important. Often, the drug given is not the active compound. Many drugs have more than one metabolite and sometimes the metabolites are more potent than the parent compound. Understanding how the drug is metabolized is essential for researchers to understand side effects and establish a safe treatment schedule. For example, if a drug is completely eliminated from a patient's body within a few hours, then the drug may need to be given daily or more than once weekly to maintain its effect on the tumor. Conversely, if a drug lasts in the patient's body for 3 weeks, then weekly dosing could cause drug accumulation and significant toxicities.

In order to retrieve accurate information from PK sampling, it is critical that the samples are drawn at specified times. Assays run on the plasma samples require special equipment and techniques. As such, sponsors often contract with outside laboratories to do the testing. Proper handling and shipping of the PK samples is essential to assure accuracy in the information they yield. Specific details about PK samples can be found in Chapter 10.

Because a phase I study seeks to answer only questions of safety, the **inclusion criteria** is generally broad. Patients with all types of cancers are typically eligible.

Some studies require that patients have measurable disease (something that can be seen by x-ray or CT scan). In the case of patients who may not have any evaluable disease, **tumor markers** may be followed. Generally, candidates also must have adequate kidney and liver function and minimal levels of white blood cells, hemoglobin, and platelets. It is also important that patients have minimal **performance status**, which is generally defined as being out of bed more than 50 percent of the day and personally taking care of most activities of daily living. These parameters are established in an attempt to avoid pre-existing problems that may confound the side effect profile and prohibit the patient from completing the trial.

Phase II Study

Phase II studies are designed to answer the questions of efficacy:

1. Does the drug work?
2. What cancers is it active against?

To that end, the patients enrolled in a particular study will all have the same diagnosis and, usually, the same prior therapies. For example, candidates would all have colorectal cancer that has been treated with 5-fluorouracil (5FU) only. Generally, about thirty patients are enrolled and given the same dose of the drug on the same schedule.

Interim analyses are frequently done during phase II studies. At the midpoint of the study, the sponsor may suspend enrollment to determine if any patient receiving the drug has already shown efficacy. Patients are restaged (that is, they have repeat CT scans) to determine whether their disease has remained stable, improved, or progressed. For example, if a study is designed to enroll forty patients, then after twenty patients have started the drug, enrollment will be suspended awaiting restaging. When at least one of the first twenty shows some reduction in tumor size, enrollment will be resumed. If no response is found in the first twenty, the study is terminated. If at least one patient shows even a partial response, the study continues and the remaining twenty patients are enrolled.

At the end of the study, the number of patients who have either stable or improved status determines the percentage of efficacy. For example, if six out of thirty patients showed either stable disease or some reduction in tumor burden or size, then the drug would be said to have 20 percent efficacy for that particular disease. Balancing the efficacy against a side effect profile defines the cost-benefit ratio of the drug.

Phase III Study

In phase III, the new therapy is tested against the current standard therapy. These studies are designed to enroll a large number of patients (600–700) and are always conducted at multiple cancer centers (50–100).

A homogeneous group of patients is randomly divided between two **arms**, one treating the patients with the standard therapy and the other treating the patients with the new therapy. For example, the study might enroll six hundred patients with untreated colorectal cancer. Three hundred of the patients would be treated with 5FU alone and the other three hundred would receive the experimental therapy. Because the study is **randomized**, patients do not have a choice of which treatment they will receive. Sometimes, everyone involved in a study except the pharmacist is **blinded**; that is, no one but the pharmacist actually knows which treatment the patient is receiving. The purpose of blinding a study is to prevent bias.

At the end of the phase III study, responses in each arm are evaluated and compared to determine whether the new therapy has an improved response rate over the standard treatment. Results of phase III trials help to define the specific indication for the drug (for example, first line or refractory to other therapy) when applying to the FDA for approval.

Often in a phase III study, **quality-of-life** questionnaires are part of the data collection. Patients are asked to complete a series of questions about their activities, pain, and perceptions of their daily functioning. Typically, the first questionnaire is completed at the baseline, before drug treatment begins, and then again at various intervals during the study. The information is then reviewed to determine whether the treatment causes a qualitative improvement in the patient's life. A drug that can improve the quality of a patient's life, even if it does not prolong it, is considered a favorable outcome. The FDA has given approval to some cancer drugs on that basis alone.

Phase IV Study

Phase IV studies are postmarketing studies initiated after the drug is commercially available. They are generally done to look at other possible uses (off-label uses) for the drug and to further assess toxicities.

Data Collection

Sponsors of the studies receive information about the progress of the trial via data collection. The importance of accurate data collection cannot be overstated. Noting everything that the patient experiences while in the trial and determining the relationship of these experiences to the study drug is essential in defining the side effects and possible toxicities of the study drug or combination of drugs. Accurate PK sampling is required to determine how the drug is metabolized. Errors either in data collection or recording could compromise patient safety and render the entire study worthless.

The sponsor provides **case report forms** (CRFs) to each study site. The forms, compiled in a book, contain information about the patients (for example, vital signs, laboratory work, concomitant medications, and adverse events). Specifics about the drug administration, including preparation time, and stop and start times, are also recorded. All data collected help researchers better understand the study drug.

Periodically, the sponsor sends out a **monitor** to review the study data against **source documentation**, or the patient's medical record. If there are discrepancies (and there always are), corrections are made.

A copy of the CRF is then pulled by the monitor and sent on to a company hired by the sponsor that enters the data into an electronic database. If during that process, missing data or other discrepancies are found, a **query** is then generated. All queries are sent back to the trial site for further correction or clarification. When the objectives of the study have been satisfied and all of the data have been reviewed and corrected, the study is officially closed. (See Part IV for a detailed discussion of this process.)

References

1. American Cancer Society, Inc. (2000). *Cancer facts & figures 2000.* Atlanta, GA, 1–3, 15, 28–32.
2. Centers for Disease Control and Prevention. (1997). Cigarette smoking: Attributable mortality and years of potential life lost—United States, 1984. *Morbidity and mortality weekly report 46,* 444–450.
3. Groenwald, S., Frogge, M., Goodman, M., & Yarbro, C. (1997). *Cancer nursing: Principles and practice 4e.* Sudbury, MA: Jones and Bartlett.
4. Nordenberg, T. (1997). Why should FDA regulate drugs? *FDA consumer,* 19–22.

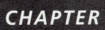

CHAPTER 2

The Protocol Process

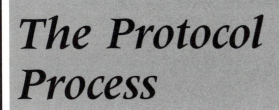

■ Understanding the Protocol

Most clinical trial protocols follow a standard format. Found within the text of the protocol are the purpose of the clinical trial, the rationale for the trial, a limited summary of the preclinical data, trial objectives, inclusion/exclusion criteria for participants, screening and study procedures, and numerous appendixes that define everything from required laboratory tests to the toxicity criteria.

The protocol is received in its final form by the principal investigator. Included is a signature page that the investigator must sign and return to the sponsor to confirm receipt. A copy of this signed page *must* be placed in the regulatory binder.

It's a good idea to make several copies of the protocol and then to disseminate the protocol to departments that will be involved in its execution, specifically the investigational pharmacy and treatment area. Exactly who should receive the protocol is determined by institutional policies and procedures.

The protocol should be read carefully with highlighter and pen in hand. After you have read and executed many protocols, this process will become much easier. However, for the first few protocols you read, it is tedious and sometimes confusing.

The Title Page

As you might expect, the title page of the protocol states the proto-col's official title. Protocol titles can sometimes be quite long and unwieldy. Consider this example:

A Phase I, Dose-Escalating, and Pharmacokinetic, Single-Center Study of ABC123, Administered Intravenously Twice Weekly for 4 Weeks, Followed by a 2-Week Rest, to Patients with All Advanced Solid Tumor Malignancies

Clearly, the title provides a lot of information. Examining each part individually, we learn the following:

1. The study is a phase I study, meaning that it is intended to answer questions of safety.
2. The study will involve dose escalation, so familiarization with the study's dose-escalation scheme will be important.
3. Pharmacokinetic (PK) sampling will be done.
4. Only one center will participate in the study.
5. The study drug will be given intravenously.
6. The study drug will be administered two times each week for 4 weeks, followed by a 2-week period without drug.
7. The cycle is 6 weeks in length.
8. The target population will be patients with all solid tumor cancers.

The protocol title also suggests questions that you will want to answer as you read the protocol. Jot your questions down for handy reference. The questions that come to mind for this example include:

- What is the dose-escalation scheme?
- How many PK samples are required, and what is the PK schedule?
- What are the requirements of IV administration?
- Does the patient need a central venous access line?
- How long will the infusion take?
- How many 6-week cycles will be done before restaging?
- Do subjects need to have measurable disease, or can patients be followed by tumor markers only?

Let's look at another example of a protocol title:

A Phase III, Randomized Study of 5FU and Leucovorin Versus 5FU and Leuco-vorin with XYZ789 for Patients with Untreated Metastatic Colorectal Cancer

Examine each part of the title, then try to answer these questions:

- What is this study designed to do?
- Can you tell from the title whether this is a standard phase III design?
- Who is the targeted patient population?
- What will you tell patients about their treatment on this protocol?

How did you do? Are you confident in your answers? Let's review the title together one more time. From the title, we learn that this is a standard phase III design that will compare the standard of care for colorectal cancer (5-fluorouracil [5FU] and leucovorin) to that same treatment plus the experimental drug XYZ789. Eligible patients will have colorectal cancer with no previous treatment. Patients who have had adjuvant therapy following surgical resection for the treatment of their disease will also be eligible. The study will be randomized, so patients cannot choose which arm of the study they will receive. When they sign the consent form, therefore, some patients will be randomized to the standard of care and will not receive the experimental treatment.

As you can see, much information can be gleaned from just the protocol title (Figure 2–1). The remainder of the title page provides the sponsor's protocol number; the IND, or investigational new drug, number, which is the investigational number given to the drug by the FDA; the name of the sponsor; and the date this version of the protocol was written. (See *Federal Regulations and Guidelines, 21 CFR 312*,[1] for U.S. Food and Drug Administration guidelines for Investigational New Drug Applications.)

A confidentiality statement is also included on the title page. Protocols are always proprietary and confidential. Copies of protocols should be made available only to those people directly involved in the execution of the protocol. For example, if a referring physician requests a copy of the protocol, the request must be denied. It is permissible to release inclusion/exclusion criteria and a short information sheet but not the entire protocol.

Information Sheets

Preparing an information sheet for a clinical trial is smart planning. Information sheets fall under the guise of advertising and must be approved by the **institutional review board** (IRB). Therefore, it is wise to prepare such documents while compiling your other IRB documents. By including the information sheet in the original submission packet, you can use them to actively recruit subjects once IRB approval has been received. See Figure 2–2for a sample information sheet. (See Chapter 3 for more on the IRB.)

PROTOCOL

TITLE: A Phase I, Dose-Escalating, and Pharmacokinetic, Single-Center Study of ABC123, Administered Intravenously Twice Weekly for 4 Weeks Followed by a 2-Week Rest to Patients with All Advanced Solid Tumor Malignancies

PROTOCOL NUMBER: ABC123.008

STUDY DRUG: ABC123

IND: 54,321

SPONSOR: The Drug Company
124 Miracle Drive
Eutopia, CA 90001
Phone: 800-555-1234
Fax: 800-555-2345

STUDY MONITOR: The Monitoring Company
100 Query Circle
Clearinfo, TX 78200
Phone: 800-222-6789
Fax: 800-222-3333

DATE OF PROTOCOL: June 15, 2000

CONFIDENTIALITY STATEMENT

Information in this protocol should not be disclosed, other than to those involved in the execution or ethical review of the study, without the written authorization from The Drug Company, Inc. It is, however, permissible to provide information to a patient in order to obtain consent.

Figure 2–1 Sample protocol title page

INFORMATION SHEET

A Phase I, dose-escalating study of ABC123 is being conducted at The Research Center under the direction of Dr. Find A. Cure. This is a single-center study for patients with all advanced solid tumor malignancies. The study drug will be given intravenously twice each week for 4 weeks, followed by 2 weeks without the drug.

ABC123 is a new class of drug that is believed to work by blocking the tumor cell receptors that allow the cell to receive growth hormones. It is believed that if a cell cannot continue to grow, it will assume the normal cell cycle and die. In animal studies, at doses much higher than those expected to be given in this study, mild hair thinning and diarrhea were seen. The study is planned to include thirty patients.

In order to be eligible, subjects must have adequate liver and renal function as well as hemoglobin greater than 9 without the use of transfusion or erythropoietin. Subjects must spend at least 50 percent of their day out of bed and be able to provide for their own needs, such as eating and dressing. It is the responsibility of the patient to obtain appropriate insurance referrals to participate in this study.

If you are interested in receiving more information about this study, please visit our Web site at www.researchcenter.org or call 1-800-555-1234.

Figure 2–2 Sample information sheet

Getting the Basics

Summary Page

In some protocols, summary page(s) are included that provide the rationale for the study, a brief description of the study drug with results of earlier trials, if applicable, and a brief synopsis of the current protocol.

Contents

A table of contents that lists each section of the protocol and the page on which it can be found is always included. Refer to the contents whenever you need to find a specific piece of information in the protocol. It's much easier than leafing through the entire protocol.

List of Abbreviations

Some protocols include a list of abbreviations to help ensure clarity. For example, PR might mean partial response or per rectum—a significant difference!

Background and Objectives

After the preliminaries comes the background, which typically begins with a statement of the problem, that is, the incidence, prevalence, and survival statistics of the targeted disease(s). Current treatment regimens are then discussed and the responses to the different regimens noted.

The study drug is then discussed in depth with attention paid to the chemistry of the compound and the animal and laboratory data (in vivo and in vitro information). Summaries of earlier studies are also reviewed. This all leads to the rationale for this particular study. Don't overload your brain to understand all of the scientific nuances of the study. Leave that to the scientists. However, you should be able to understand the basics of how the drug works. If you don't, talk to someone who can explain it to you.

Following the rationale, the primary and secondary objectives of the study are stated. Be sure that you understand the specific goals of the study, and keep them in mind as you read the rest of the protocol; are you looking at tumor response, time to progression, or time to survival? You may, in fact, be looking for all of that information, but be sure you understand the primary objective.

Inclusion and Exclusion Criteria

Who is your study population? What are the inclusion criteria, and what are the exclusion criteria? You will be expected to know this information inside and out. Answers to the inclusion questions must be YES, and answers to the exclusion questions must be NO. Read each item carefully and be sure that you understand *exactly* what conditions the patient must meet in order to be eligible for this study. Consider reducing the inclusion/exclusion criteria page on a photocopier to a convenient size, so you can carry it in your pocket as a quick reference when you are in clinic. If you are responsible for several protocols, remembering details of the inclusion or exclusion criteria for each protocol is not humanly possible.

If you have a good candidate for the study, but there is one minor problem that excludes him or her, you might decide to ask the sponsor for an **exception**. For example, an otherwise excellent candidate for the study may have had a superficial skin cancer removed 3 years prior. If the exclusion criteria excludes individuals who have had a cancer within 5 years, an exception will be needed to get the patient enrolled. Send an e-mail to the medical monitor, a physician employed by the sponsor, who is responsible for clinical decisions. Give the patient's initials, date of birth, and disease, as well as the exact section of the protocol that requires the exclusion. Be sure to indicate why the principal investigator believes an exception should be granted. Send the request promptly, and allow sufficient time for the sponsor to review and respond to the request. The sponsor may ask for additional information, such as the pathology report in this case.

If an exception is requested and granted, you should indicate this on the registration form when you send it to the sponsor. In turn, the sponsor should send a formal letter, signed by the medical monitor, officially granting the exception. File the original letter in the regulatory binder under "study correspondence." Place one copy in the case report form (CRF) with the patient's registration, and another in the patient's research chart.

It is wise to confirm any conversation you have had with the study personnel via e-mail and then to file hard copy of the document in both the regulatory binder and the CRF. Exceptions given by the sponsor may need to be reported to your IRB (see Chapter 3 for more information).

Study Procedures

The study procedures provide essential information for the study coordinator, outlining *exactly* what must be done to screen the patient, the baseline studies required, and the intrastudy procedures. Pay careful attention to the date requirements (Figure 2–3). Concomitant therapies that are allowed and disallowed, dose modifications/delays, and drug administration are discussed; the criteria for termination from the study are outlined. Read this section carefully because the criteria may differ from study to study. Consider making copies of this information to keep in a binder. It will save you a lot of running around to find answers in the middle of a busy clinic.

Most studies require follow-up with patients 30 days after stopping the study drug, and every few months thereafter, for survival information. Usually, the 30-day follow-up requires a physical examination and lab work. Further follow-ups are generally done by a phone call. This process may vary from protocol to protocol, so note these requirements.

Adverse Events

Adverse events (AE) and serious adverse events (SAE) are thoroughly discussed. Basically, any change that occurs after the patient has started the study drug is called an **adverse event**. You must clearly distinguish between symptoms present at **baseline** and what is new. For example, if the patient had shoulder pain at the screening visit, shoulder pain would only be an adverse event if it increased in intensity

DATE REQUIREMENTS

Study Procedures

1. Screening Procedures

To be conducted **within 28 days prior to initiating therapy**, except where noted.

1.1 Patient or legally authorized representative must understand and sign Informed Consent Form prior to any protocol-related examination or procedures.

1.2 A complete medical history will be obtained, including history of malignancy, history of treatment for malignancy, and notation of concomitant medications.

1.3 **Within 14 days prior to initiating therapy**, tumor assessment (radiographic measurement, serum tumor marker or physical clinical measurement) will be undertaken to document the extent of the disease.

1.4 **Within 7 days prior to initiating therapy**, a complete physical examination, including vital signs, height, weight, performance status, and a list of current symptoms will occur.

1.5 **Within 7 days prior to initiating therapy**, samples for serum chemistry, hematology, coagulation studies, and urinalysis will be obtained.

1.6 **Within 7 days prior to initiating therapy**, all at-risk female patients (not surgically sterile or postmenopausal) must have a serum pregnancy test.

Figure 2–3 Date requirements

or changed in character. Understanding adverse events will be discussed in more depth in Chapter 11.

Serious adverse events have specific criteria that are discussed in Chapter 11, under Data Collection. The verbiage used to describe SAEs in protocols is fairly standard. Serious adverse events must be reported to both the sponsor and the IRB within a specified time period. Be sure that you know the requirements.

Statistics

There is specific information about the statistical analysis of the data that is great for a statistician. Do not worry about getting this in full, leave that to the sponsor and the IRB.

What you need to understand is that your population, or the number of subjects enrolled in the study, is designated by n. If 40 subjects are enrolled in the study, $n = 40$. A statistician determines the number of subjects to be enrolled in the study to ensure a statistically significant outcome.

Appendices

Many appendices are included with the protocol. The schedule of events is usually the first; you will refer to it often. This page is another good candidate for copying and will prove an invaluable reference. Other appendices outline specifics relating to various study criteria and might include, for example, a scale for determining a patient's performance status, handling and shipping of pharmacokinetic samples, toxicity criteria (either National Cancer Institute [NCI] or World Health Organization [WHO]), and drug supply, distribution, and accountability information.

■ *Really* Understanding the Protocol

After reading the protocol once, you will have a fair understanding of what the study will be like. Many of your initial questions may have been answered, but now you may have new questions. Read the protocol again, skipping the background, scientific, and statistical parts if you wish. In this pass, you will find even more answers and probably a few more questions. Then read the protocol again, formulating in your mind and on paper how it should be executed. Continue rereading the protocol until you gain a clear understanding of it. If some things remain unclear, make notes and pose your questions at the **investigators' meeting** or the **site initiation visit**. Not every protocol is perfectly written!

You may want to place tabs or flags on pages of the protocol that you will refer to frequently. Consider marking the inclusion/exclusion criteria, the screening procedures, the study requirements within each cycle, and the end of study pages. You will read and reread these pages over and over again as you begin screening and treating patients. Using tabs eliminates the frustration of trying to find something specific in a hurry.

◼ Reference

1. Federal Regulations and Guidelines. *Code of federal regulations, 1998.* 21 CFR 312.

CHAPTER 3

Regulatory Issues

◼ Institutional Review Board

Before a center can begin to accrue patients, the protocol must be submitted to the organization's institutional review board (IRB) for review and approval. The institutional review board seeks to protect the rights of individuals who enroll in a study.

The Need for the IRB

In the late 1900s, great industries began to arise. The Government supported the growth of business, and any social change to benefit that growth was acceptable. By the turn of the century, it was clear that legislation was needed to safeguard the interests of citizens worldwide. In 1906, Upton Sinclair published his now classic novel, *The Jungle,* which exposed unsanitary meat handling in Chicago's slaughterhouses.[1] Although seen as propaganda at the time, the book spurred passage of the Food and Drug Law of 1906 requiring food purity. Further legislation came in response to an elixir of sulfanilamide, marketed by the Massengill Drug Company, that killed 107 people. The Food, Drug, and Cosmetic Drug Act of 1938 was the first law to require that companies establish drug safety prior to marketing a compound.

The Declaration of Helsinki, which is internationally recognized as a worldwide standard in clinical trials, was issued in Finland in 1961.[2] The declaration addresses standards for medical personnel in research with human subjects. The U.S. Public Health Service mandated use of IRBs and issued regulations for informed consent involving human research subjects in 1966.

In the early 1960s, thalidomide, a drug intended to control the nausea and vomiting associated with early pregnancy, was tested. Between 1960 and 1961, more than 300 infants were born with birth defects resulting from their mother's use of thalidomide. In 1962, the Kefauver-Harris Amendments to the Food, Drug, and Cosmetic Act required companies to establish the efficacy of their products, as well as adhere to new requirements with regards to purity and safety, *before* making them available to the public. The Act also required that research subjects give **informed consent** before they could be treated with an experimental drug. Other amendments included requirements for use of accurate and ethical advertising to recruit subjects.

Ethics and the IRB

The ethics of clinical trials came into unfavorable focus when, in 1972, an account of the Tuskegee Syphilis Study sparked public outrage. In 1932, the U.S. Public Health Service began a study of syphilis in black men in the small, rural town of Tuskegee, Alabama. The purpose of the study was to determine the natural course of syphilis in adult, black men. The control group included 200 men without syphilis; the study group included 400 men with untreated syphilis. Even though penicillin was then known to be an effective treatment for syphilis, the men were not treated. In fact, deliberate steps were taken to keep the subjects from receiving treatment.

It was later determined that information had been withheld from study participants. Many did not understand the purpose of the study, nor did some realize they were participating in a study. Reports of the study were published as early as 1936, but no action was taken to stop it. Even as late as 1969, the Centers for Disease Control believed that the study should continue. Finally, after the public outrage of 1972, the Department of Health, Education and Welfare stopped the study.[3]

In 1978, The National Commission for the Protection of Human Subjects of Biomedical and Behavioral Research examined the issue of human experimentation and explored its ethical and human rights implications. The commission's findings and recommendations were published in the Belmont Report, which established stricter guidelines for the information provided to research subjects.[4] The goal was to promote greater respect for an individual's autonomy and give more attention to beneficence and justice for all humans involved in clinical trials. The report addressed the need for documentation in the informed consent form of the risks versus benefits of a clinical trial and also set guidelines for special protection for children and the mentally ill.

You will frequently hear reference to Good Clinical Practice (GCP). Good Clinical Practice is an international ethical and scientific quality standard for designing, conducting, recording, and reporting clinical trials that involve the participation of human subjects. The origin of this guideline is the Declaration of Helsinki (1961); GCP provides public assurance that the rights, safety, and well-being of participants in clinical trials are protected. The objective of the GCP is to provide a unified standard of practice for the European Union (EU), Japan, and the United States in order to facilitate the mutual acceptance of clinical data by the regulatory authorities in those jurisdictions.[5] The guidelines were last updated in May 1997 as a result of the International Conference on Harmonisation (ICH).

Institutional review boards vary from institution to institution, and their filing procedures also vary widely. Some IRBs are informal, requiring a minimal amount of paperwork; others require many forms and a rigorous review of all information. FDA guidelines for the protection of human subjects and for institutional review boards can be found in the Federal Regulations and Guidelines, 21 CFR 50 and 21 CFR 56, respectively.[6]

Regardless of the type of IRB, you will be expected to submit to the board a copy or copies of the current protocol, the **investigator's brochure**, a statement of financial disclosure from the principal investigator, and a copy of the informed consent. Many IRBs also have forms that require specific questions be answered; for example, What are your recruiting procedures? Because the membership of the IRB is a combination of scientific, medical, and laypeople, the board often requests a summary of the protocol written in layman's language.

■ Informed Consent

Informed consent has been a hot topic for years and will likely always be so. Volumes have been written about informed consent, the patient's right to know, and the patient's bill of rights, among others. Indeed, each of these issues is extremely important. How much detail an informed consent must include is often driven by an institution's IRB. For example, at some institutions, it does not suffice to say that the patient will have certain blood tests. Instead, the amount of blood to be drawn must be stated in layman's terms, that is, in teaspoons or tablespoons.

Clarity of Language

The most important issue about writing an informed consent is that it must be in language the patient can understand. Using language, which does not exceed the eighth-grade reading level is appropriate. You need to remember that even if IV is a term that is very common-place to you, you must assume that it is not to the patient. Therefore, you will need to explain IV as "through a needle in your vein" in the consent form.

Level of Detail

Concerns about liability and the patient's right to know have prompted consent forms that are ten to twenty pages long. Undoubt-edly, there will always be patients who absorb every word and still want more information, as well as patients who are overwhelmed just in looking at a document that looks that formal. FDA guidelines of 1995 allow the use of shorter consent forms, but most IRBs continue to advocate detailed consent forms to guarantee that patients are fully informed.

Need for Translation

Recruiting patients from varied ethnic backgrounds causes special problems, as it is impossible to accurately anticipate the need for con-sent forms in translation. Although a patient may be consented with a translator present, he or she also must receive a translated copy of the consent form to sign. This process can be costly in terms of time required and actual expense. (See Chapter 4.)

Late Details and Revisions

During the course of a clinical trial, new information may arise. For example, some patients may experience an unanticipated cough that may be related to the drug. Such information must be communicated to the patients currently in the trial, and a revised consent form must be written. The revised consent must again be approved by the IRB, and then all patients in the study must be reconsented.

Over the course of a study, many revisions to the consent form may be needed. When a new patient enrolls, he or she must sign the current consent form. Likewise, patients who have been in the study for an extended period of time may have several iterations of the consent form in their records.

Preparing a Consent Form

Most consents are required to address the following areas of importance.

Purpose of the Study

This information should be taken from the objectives stated in the protocol.

Procedures Involved in Participating in the Study

Identify, step-by-step, what is involved from the first screening visit through the follow-up visit after study termination. This section should include information about all blood tests, EKGs, CT scans, physical examinations, and anything else the patient will be asked to do during the course of the study.

Potential Risks and Discomforts

All possible side effects must be outlined in this section. Consult the investigator's brochure for information gleaned from previous animal and human trials if applicable. In addition to describing what is known about the drug, note that previously unknown side effects may occur, even death. The risk of pregnancy is also discussed with the statement that patients must also agree to use adequate methods of contraception because effects of the drug(s) on unborn fetuses are not known.

Potential Benefits

This is usually a brief statement of what benefits have already been seen in animal and/or human trials with a caveat that the drug(s) may be of no benefit at all to the patient. A statement about the potential contribution of participation to other people or future research can also be made here.

Alternative to Participation

Other alternatives to participation in this trial from no treatment or best supportive care to conventional therapies are briefly discussed in this section.

Compensation for Participation

Note here if the patient is to be paid for participation in the trial. If so, how much and when payment will be made must be stated.

Financial Obligation

This is a section that always evokes questions. In general, the study drug, its administration, and all tests that are specifically related to the experimental nature of the study are provided or paid for by the study's sponsor. Blood tests and other procedures that are normally part of the care of a patient being treated for the particular disease can and should be billed to insurance. If a patient normally pays 20 percent of all medical bills, then the patient should expect to pay 20 percent of all costs that are billed to the insurance company.

In this day of managed care, treating patients who are part of a health maintenance organization (HMO) becomes extremely complicated. All issues must be carefully discussed in detail prior to the patient signing the consent. If authorizations are required by the HMO, everyone must understand what authorizations are needed, when they must be secured, and who is responsible for obtaining them.

Emergency Care and Compensation for Injury

If the patient is injured as a result of participation in the study, the sponsor is expected to pay for the patient's treatment. However, here it is customary to make a statement indemnifying the participating medical institution from liability.

Confidentiality

Patients should be assured that their identities will remain confidential. Although information about their treatment and response will be shared with the sponsor, the FDA, the IRB, and the researchers participating in the study, every effort will be made to guarantee the patient's privacy. Incorporating a statement here about needing to obtain records of previous treatment from other institutions allows use of this page and the signature page to obtain any needed outside records.

Participation and Withdrawal

State that participation in the study is voluntary to begin this section. State also that the patient may withdraw consent at any time. Outline the conditions under which continued participation is allowed, that is, if the disease does not progress, if there are no severe toxicities, if the patient complies with study requirements, and if the study is not discontinued.

New Findings

State that if any new information is obtained, good or bad, the patient will be informed.

Identification of Investigators

The principal investigator and all of the subinvestigators should be named, and their addresses, telephone numbers, and emergency numbers are provided.

Rights of Research Subjects

Here, revisit the patient's right to withdraw consent at any time. Also, supply the name, address, and telephone number of the IRB in case the patient has any questions about his or her rights.

Signature Page

State briefly that the patient has read and understands all of the information in the consent form and acknowledges receipt of a copy of the consent. It is best to provide a line for the patient to print his or her name, then a line for the signature followed by the date and time. The FDA requires that consent be obtained prior to any screening procedures. If screening is being done on the same day consent is secured, then the time will indicate whether the FDA guideline has been met.

Although only the patient's signature is required on the consent, many institutions require that the document be countersigned by the investigator or the designee who has explained the consent. Date and time should follow this signature as well.

If the patient is a minor or has a guardian, or needs a translator, then the guardian or translator also needs to sign the consent, indicating the relationship or role in the consenting process as well as the date and time of signature. (See Chapter 8 for a discussion of obtaining consent.)

Consent Approval

Once the consent form is written, the sponsor must review it to ensure that their regulatory people are in agreement with all statements *before* the consent is submitted to the IRB. There may be conflicts between what the sponsor feels comfortable stating in the consent and what the IRB requires for resolution. The principal investigator and the medical monitor or their legal counsel may need to confer.

When both sides are in agreement, submit the consent to the IRB for approval. Always prepare the consent on a computer disk so that text changes can be made easily. It may take more than one pass through the IRB before final approval is granted.

■ Form 1572

Form 1572 is required by the FDA and lists the investigators involved in the particular clinical trial. In addition to naming the principal investigator and coinvestigators, the form includes the names of participating laboratories, their current addresses, and information about where to ship the drug. If new laboratories are added during the trial, a new Form 1572 must be generated. All Form 1572s must be signed, a copy sent to the sponsor, and the original filed in the regulatory binder.

■ Statement of Economic Interest

If the principal investigator owns stock, sits on an advisory board, or have some economic interest in the sponsor, this information must be disclosed to the IRB. The main purpose of this report is to assure that investigators are not biased in recruiting subjects or reporting of information about the subjects or the study drug. In the near future, *all* parties involved in conducting the study, including coinvestigators, study coordinators and data managers, may also be required to complete statements of economic interest.

■ Lay Language Summary

Many IRBs require a synopsis of the protocol in layman's language. The purpose of the summary is to assist nonmedical members of the IRB committee to gain a quick overview of the protocol in language that is easily understood.

■ Regulatory Binder

The sponsor provides a notebook, called the regulatory binder, which is the official file for the study.

When a protocol is first received from the sponsor, the principal investigator signs an acknowledgment of receipt and returns the original to the sponsor. A copy of the acknowledgment and all original Form 1572s are filed in the regulatory binder. Typically, regulatory binders are organized as follows.

Protocol

All versions of the protocol used throughout the study are filed here. For example, if the protocol is amended three times before the study is completed, four separate protocols will be filed under this section.

Informed Consent

All informed consents and addenda to the consents are filed here. Signed copies of all of the investigators' curriculum vitae (CV) and licenses must be included in the binder and updated when renewed or at least yearly. Any laboratories that are used during the trial must submit the laboratory's certification, license, and lab normals, which are filed in the binder as well. Laboratory certifications include CLIA (Clinical Laboratory Improvement Amendments) and CAP (College of American Pathologists). The CLIAs and CAPs must be updated yearly.

Record-Keeping Suggestion

Consider creating a simple log to track when CVs and CLIAs expire, as a trigger for requesting new licenses. When a new license is received, enter it in the log, and continue this process for the duration of the study (Table 3–1).

During the study, a patient may request to have required labs done at another facility. Most sponsors will allow the variance provided the CLIA and lab norms are obtained from the outside facility and its name and address are added to the Form 1572.

IRB Documents

All outgoing or incoming communication with the IRB must be filed in this section. Submissions, approval letters, updates, renewals, and reports of all serious adverse events (SAEs) reside here. Protocols must be renewed annually while patients are actively participating in the study. All requests for renewal and letters of approval *must* be filed in this section of the regulatory binder. The sponsor must also receive file copies of all approvals.

Study Correspondence

Correspondence with the sponsor is filed in this section. If communication occurs via e-mail, print a hard copy of the document

Table 3–1 Sample License Log			
License	Expiration Date	New License Requested	New License Received
Dr. F. A. Cure	11/99	11/1/99	11/15/99
Special Lab	1/00		
Dr. F. A. Cure	11/00		

and include it here. Document all significant phone conversations completely to ensure thorough records. To avoid misunderstandings, document phone conversations by e-mail and file the hard copy here.

Tracking Logs

Within the binder there are several tracking logs. The *screening log* lists all patients screened for the study. Patients are identified by initials and date of birth; the patient's status—whether enrolled or not—is also recorded. If the patient was not enrolled, an explanation why the patient failed screening is noted. It is important to keep this log updated because it shows the sponsor that you are making an effort to accrue to the study, even if enrollment is low. In studies that have difficulty accruing patients, the information on this log may identify a need to amend the protocol.

The *patient tracking log* documents each patient visit by date. This log helps sponsors track patients in the study; sponsors often request that this log be faxed weekly.

Signature Log

Every investigator in the study and everyone who writes in the case report form (CRF) must sign the signature log.

Delegation of Authority Form

The principal investigator must delegate responsibilities to a variety of personnel during the course of the study. Clearly, he or she cannot personally oversee every aspect of a study. Therefore, a Delegation of Authority Form has become a part of the regulatory documents. This form defines the roles of all personnel within the research team for the sponsor and the FDA in case of an audit. Additionally, the form illustrates each person's signature, initials, and how he or she writes each number, 0 through 9 (Figure 3–1).

Although the principal investigator may delegate certain functions to others on the team, that does not negate his or her responsibility. It is important to document that the team members report to the investigator on a regular basis. For example, the investigator may hold a weekly team meeting during which all delegated aspects of the protocol are discussed. A copy of the minutes of those meetings should be available for review upon request.

Designing a form to use to report on each patient is a valuable tool; see Figure 3–2. This form should be updated weekly prior to the team meeting and any comment such as CTs pending, or ↑LFTs (liver

Delegation of Authority Form

Protocol Number: _____

Investigator: _____

Center: _____

INVESTIGATOR'S AUTHORIZATION: I hereby delegate the following trial-related duties to the persons listed below. The overall responsibility for the conduct of the trial remains with me.

Full Name	Title and Position	Initials and Signature with Date	Write the Numbers 0 1 2 3 4 5 6 7 8 9	Authorization Codes	Investigator's Signature with Date

Authorization Codes:

1 = Informed Consent Discussion
2 = Perform Physical Examination
3 = Interview the Patient re: Adverse Events

4 = CRF Entries
5 = Prescribe Drugs
6 = Drug Dispensation

7 = Drug Administration
8 = Drug Reconciliation
9 = Other (specify)

Figure 3–1 Delegation of authority form (CRF = case report form)

ABC 123 Patient List

Principal Investigator: Find A. Cure, MD

Study Coordinator: Inta Detail, RN

Patient Name	Patient Initials	Study Number	Sex	Ethnicity	Date Accrued	Date First Treated	Tx Course	Date Off Study	Referring MD	Site MD	Comments
Screened											
Active											
Off Study											
Screen Failed											

Figure 3–2 Patient list

function tests), can be added as a reminder of pertinent information on a specific patient.

This form can have many uses outside of your team. If your institution requires reporting of patient accrual and gender and ethnicity to a specific department, sending a copy of the report meets that requirement without generating another report. If the finance department wants to know on study and off study dates for each patient, putting them on the distribution list will cover that need. The list can even serve as a screening and enrollment log for the sponsor.

As you can guess, by the end of a study the binder generally becomes multiple binders many volumes. To keep the regulatory binder current, simply file every form or letter when it arrives. In that way, nothing will get lost. The study monitor will check the regulatory binder at each visit.

■ References

1. Sinclair, U. (1906). *The jungle.* New York: Doubleday, Page & Company.
2. International Conference on Harmonisation. (1997). *Good clinical practices: Consolidated guideline: notice of availability.* Federal Register, 62 (90).
3. McCarthy, C. R. (1994). Historical background of clinical trials involving women and minorities. *Academic Medicine,* 69, 695–698.
4. National Commission for the Protection of Human Subjects of Biomedical and Behavioral Research. (1978). *The Belmont report.* DHEW Publication No. (05)78.0013 and No. (05)78.0014. USGPO, Washington, D.C.
5. International Conference on Harmonisation; *Good clinical practice: consolidated guideline; availability* (1997). Federal Register, 62(90).
6. Federal Regulations and Guidelines. *Code of federal regulations.* (1996). Federal Register, 61(192).

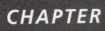
The Budget

■ Understanding the Basic Expenses

Writing a budget for a clinical trial can be fairly easy with a little knowledge and practice. Finding a balance between covering costs, including the salaries of research personnel, and remaining competitive with other research centers is key.

Don't attempt the budgeting process until you have read the protocol several times and have a good understanding of what will be needed to execute the trial. When you are ready to begin budgeting, read the protocol again, with your financial hat on. Note the frequency of blood tests, physician visits, pharmacokinetic sampling, EKGs, radiographic examinations, and anything that is ordered to answer purely experimental questions. It is prudent to extract this information from the text of the protocol and then to compare it with the study schedule, looking for possible discrepancies. If the study schedule and the information in the protocol are consistent, work from the study schedule. However, the study schedule may not define the frequency of PK sampling and you may need to refer to the text of the protocol for that information.

In order to determine what should be part of the budget, it is first necessary to establish what insurance companies consider normal and customary. Table 4–1 gives a breakdown of some of the common tests

Table 4–1	Customary Insurance Charges
Activity or Test	**Frequency Allowed**
Physician's visit	Monthly
Complete blood count, differential and platelets	Weekly
Chemistry panel	Monthly
EKG	Baseline
Urinalysis	Monthly
Chest x-ray	Monthly
CT scans	Every 8–12 weeks
PT, APTT	Baseline
Tumor markers	Monthly

PT = prothrombin time; APTT = activated partial thromboplastin time.

and the frequency that insurance companies consider customary. If the protocol asks for physician visits only once every month, for example, then all physician visits can be billed directly to the patient's insurance. Likewise, weekly CBCs would be billed to the patient's insurance. If the protocol asks for a weekly chemistry panel during a 4-week cycle, however, then the sponsor will be obligated to pay for three of the four chemistry panels.

Any test that is not usually required for a patient with cancer should also be considered part of the expected reimbursement by the sponsor. Laboratory tests, such as flow cytometry, amylase, or creatinine phosphokinase (CPK), that are being drawn to monitor something specific about the study compound must be billed to the sponsor via the budget.

If a patient is participating in an experimental protocol, the insurance company should reimburse for the normal and customary costs that would otherwise be paid if the patient were receiving another form of cancer treatment. In some states, it has been made illegal for insurance companies to refuse payment for reasonable costs associated with participation in a clinical trial. Recently, the National Cancer Institute (NCI) reported results of a study in which costs were compared for 270 patients who entered cancer clinical trials at Kaiser Permanente in northern California. The patients were equally divided, one-half enrolled in clinical trials and the other half enrolled as a control group. The study concluded that participation in clinical trials at a large health maintenance organization (HMO) did not result in substantial increases in the direct costs of medical care.[1]

Managed-care companies often give limited authorization for payment if their patients participate in a clinical trial at an organization that is outside the preferred provider pool. For example, they may allow a monthly physician's visit but demand that all laboratory work and radiographic studies be done at their facility. Situations like this can become incredibly challenging for the study coordinator. When such work is done outside the host facility, it is difficult to ensure that the correct tests are being done, and sometimes next to impossible to have the results faxed promptly.

■ Determining Your Costs

Most departments within your organization will provide a discounted rate for their services. The amount charged within the organization will be less than what is billed to insurance. Be sure to consult with each department before you begin budgeting, so that you are working with accurate discounted rates when determining your costs. See Figure 4–1 for a sample budget proposal. As you can see, the budget is divided into three sections: fixed costs, cycle 1, and additional cycles.

Fixed Costs

Most institutional review boards (IRBs) do not charge a fee to review and approve a protocol. However, you must ensure reimbursement for the costs of preparing the IRB submission which takes a considerable amount of time. Imagine what would happen if you submitted a protocol—not considering start-up costs in the budget—and the sponsor decided to withdraw. You would have spent a lot of time, energy, and resources without any hope for reimbursement. Start-up costs, also called fixed costs, are not enrollment or cycle-dependent. They remain the same regardless of the number of patients accrued or the length of the study.

Likewise, the investigational pharmacist spends considerable time determining how the drug will be prepared and administered, and establishes what equipment will be needed (for example, IV bags, tubing, filters, and pumps). When the drug is received, it must be inventoried and shelved under the proper conditions. Pharmacy start-up costs are important considerations because, again, if the sponsor withdraws the protocol, much of the work has already been done.

If a sponsor withdraws a protocol before the contract is signed and the budget agreed to, most sponsors will reimburse your reasonable start-up costs. Sponsors will likely want to work with your institution again in the future and will, therefore, make every effort to sustain a good relationship.

Cycle 1 Costs

Cycle 1 costs include all of the screening studies that are not covered by insurance as well as specific cycle 1 costs, such as pharmacokinetic

Budget Proposal

TITLE: A Phase I Study of XYZ123 Given Weekly in the
                                      Treatment of Patients with Advanced
                                      Malignancies

IRB#:   99-08-123

PRINCIPAL INVESTIGATOR: Find A. Cure, MD
                                      New Therapy Medical Group
                                      100 Research Boulevard
                                      Cancerfree, CA 90001

GRANTOR: XYZ, Inc.
                                      123 Main Street
                                      Hoboken, NJ 00000

ITEMIZATION	FIXED COSTS	CYCLE 1*	ADDITIONAL CYCLES*
Professional Services/ MD Fees		$1,000	$ 250
Research Coordinator/ Data Management		$2,000	$ 500
IRB Set-up Fee	$1,500		
Pharmacy			
Set-up Fee (Cycle 1)	$650 (+ $350 each yr. thereafter)		
Study Drug Preparation		$ 300	$ 300
Laboratory		$ 425	$ 250
EKG		$ 100	NA
PK Samples		$ 300	$ 300
Inpatient Nursing		$ 700	$ 700
Outpatient Nursing		$ 900	$ 900
SUBTOTAL	$2,150	$5,725	$3,200
OVERHEAD 22.5%	$ 484	$1,288	$ 720
TOTAL COSTS	**$2,634**	**$7,013**	**$3,920**

This budget assumes that the insurer will pay the cost of the staging assessment at the end of every other
cycle. If not, sponsor agrees to reimburse at the discounted research cost. If other research-related studies are
needed beyond the usual insurance reimbursement, Sponsor will be billed accordingly.
*per patient

Figure 4–1 Sample budget proposal (IRB = institutional review board; NA
= not applicable; PK = pharmacokinetic)

(PK) sampling. Depending on how your institution handles PK samples, remember to consider each step required—drawing, spinning, freezing, and shipping the samples—which together can amount to a very time-consuming and costly process. When budgeting, don't be too conservative. Unforeseen or unexpected costs are a given. By allowing a small cushion in the budget, you'll be prepared to address problems as they occur without having to operate at a loss or negotiate with the sponsor over minor issues.

If a special examination or procedure is required at baseline (for example, an ophthalmological examination or flow cytometry), determine where the examination will take place, by whom, and what the cost will be. *Never* guesstimate such costs because they may be much more than you might anticipate.

Important Note

The charges for the physician's services and for the research coordinator/data management are the most negotiable numbers in the budget. These charges can provide some flexibility when budgeting if you need it. However, do not short change yourself. Remember to consider the amount of your time the patient population will need either because of the acuity of the patients or the complexity of the protocol.

Additional Cycles column of the budget reflects all expenses that must be paid for by the sponsor during each additional patient cycle. You will note that the professional fees, MD, Research Coordinator and Data Management fees, are much lower than in cycle 1. The amount of your time required during additional cycles is probably significantly less than in cycle 1; therefore, the cost is lower. However, sometimes cycle 2 can be as demanding as cycle 1 with the exception of baseline screening procedures. Read your protocol carefully to determine a fair charge for those items. You may need to design a budget which has separate columns for cycle 1, cycle 2, and then cycle 3+. The format you choose needs to be based on the protocol requirements.

Sponsor Input

The sponsor typically sends a sample budget outlining the amount that they would like to pay to the test site for each patient treated on the protocol. If the bottom line of your budget is nowhere near the sponsor's bottom line, revisit your numbers. Be certain that you and the sponsor's representative are in agreement about which tests must be done. It's possible that the sponsor's representative who is negotiating with you is not familiar with every detail of the study. For example, one representative questioned a $500 charge for EKGs. It quickly became apparent that he was not aware that the protocol called for an EKG *every week* of the 5-week cycle; he thought the $500 charge was for one EKG.

Investigator Input

When the budget approaches the sponsor's numbers, present it to the principal investigator for input. The amounts budgeted for physician services and research coordinator/data management are logical places to make adjustments. Also note in Figure 4–1 that cycle 1 fees are higher than those for subsequent cycles. A great deal of time and work is required to enroll a patient in a clinical trial. Cycle 1 also usually necessitates more visits and closer monitoring of the patient than do other cycles. Also, if a patient goes off study after only one cycle, you will want to be sure to have covered your costs.

Translation Fees

Remember the discussion about providing a copy of the informed consent to foreign-speaking patients in their native language (see Chapter 3)? Well, don't forget to research the cost of such translations, and be sure to factor that cost into the budget. If translation is not anticipated to be a frequent expense, you may want to consider invoicing the sponsor directly for each translation.

■ Unreimbursed Expenses

The costs that never get reimbursed are the hundreds of phone calls you make to screen patients who are then determined to be ineligible. Likewise, the screening costs for patients you see who are then deemed ineligible are also unreimbursed. Bear all of that in mind when you write your budget. Just be careful. Once again, do not set yourself up for a loss. If you cannot cover your costs and your salaries, the research program will not survive.

■ Overhead

One last, but costly, item. Some institutions require that a certain percentage—from 20 to 30 percent—be added to the budget for overhead. In such a budget, remember that your bottom line must include the overhead percentage. Overhead is costly and will significantly impact your budget, so be sure all of your numbers are correct before submitting the budget to the sponsor. Once the budget has been approved by the sponsor, you are usually stuck with it.

■ Award Synopsis

When the budget has been agreed to, an award synopsis is prepared and is sent with the budget·to the sponsor and financial and contract people at your institution. The per-patient cost is multiplied by the total number of patients anticipated to be enrolled during the entire study.

Fixed Costs	$ 2,634
Cycle 1 @ $7,013 × 10 patients	70,130
TOTAL	$72,764

The additional cycles would be invoiced to the sponsor at certain intervals, usually quarterly.

■ Budget Adjustments

If, during the course of the study, the sponsor adds additional work not originally outlined in the protocol, it is perfectly acceptable to write an addendum to the budget. Also, if you find that something that sounded relatively simple at the outset has turned out to be your worst nightmare and is requiring hours of your time, discuss the matter with the sponsor. The sponsor may decide that the activity or test is not really necessary or, if it is important, that you should add a few more dollars to the budget.

■ Payment Schedule

The payment schedule generally accompanies the budget. Payments can be made in many different ways. Often, fixed costs are paid when the first patient is accrued. After that, payments are made quarterly and are determined by the data that is monitored, removed (or pulled) from the case report forms (CRFs) and sent for entry into the database. For example, let's say that in the first 3 months of the study, you have enrolled ten patients. The data has been reviewed, corrected, and pulled for six of the patients through cycle 1 and also through cycle 2 for three patients. You should be paid as follows:

6 Cycle 1 @ $7,013 = $42,078
3 Cycle 2 @ $3,920 = <u>11,760</u>
TOTAL = $53,838

Alternatively, a percent of the total budget can be paid at certain patient accrual points. Such a payment schedule might look like this:

10%	Contact signed
10%	First patient accrued
30%	Five patients accrued
30%	Accrual completed
10%	Study closed
10%	Database closed

It is essential to keep track of what data have been pulled and what payments have been received. Some institutions have a fund manager to assist in this important but tedious process. Payments might be lost in the mail, credited to the wrong account, or simply not made, and without careful monitoring you could be totally unaware of payment status. Table 4–2 is a sample form that you may want to develop to track payments if you are being compensated as data are pulled.

The information in Table 4–2 tells you that at the end of the first quarter, March 30, 1999, the sponsor should be billed for cycle 1 times 3 and cycle 2 times 1. If we use the figures from the sample budget (see Figure 4–1), then the bill should be $24,959 ([$7,013 × 3] +

Table 4–2 Sample Payment Tracking Form

STUDY NAME: Phase I ABC123

Date	Patient #	Cycle #
2/13/99	1	1
2/13/99	2	1
3/15/99	3	1
3/15/99	1	2

Table 4–3 Study Cost Grid		
Activity or Test	**Insurance**	**Sponsor**
Physician visits	X	
Study drug preparation		X
Study drug administration		X
Chest x-ray	X	
PK sampling		X
CT scans	X	

PK = pharmacokinetic.

$3,920). Placing a big red line or a blank space between the quarters will help you keep track of what payment belongs in which quarter.

■ Billing Issues

Once it's been determined how each component of the study will be charged, ensure that everyone who will generate charges knows what should be billed to insurance and what should be billed to the sponsor. With the information from the budget, prepare a **study cost grid** (Table 4–3) and share it with the finance department and the treatment area. The study cost grid delineates which costs are billed to insurance and which are billed to the sponsor. Some organizations program this information into the computer to help ensure that charges are properly billed when the patients begin treatment.

When preparing requisitions or charge documents for each of the study's tests indicate on the form that the test should be billed to insurance or to the sponsor. When all financial information is in place, an account number will be assigned to the study. In order to avoid billing problems, include the account number on each requisition. For example,

Do *not* bill patient. Bill to account RCH77777-33.

No matter how much effort is expended in setting up the billing details, it's unlikely that every person in every department will do everything correctly (ever heard of Utopia?). Warn patients that billing errors occur on occasion, and instruct them to bring in for your review any bills they don't understand or that seem incorrect.

■ Reference

1. Fireman, B. H., Fehrenbacher, L., Gruskin, E. P., & Ray, G. T. (2000). Cost of care for patients in cancer clinical trials. *Journal of the National Cancer Institute*, 92 (2), 136–142.

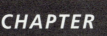

CHAPTER 5

The Contract

Although you may have little to no input in the contract negotiations, you cannot go brain dead at the sight of the contract; you must understand the process and keep track of its progress.

A **contract** is an agreement between the study site and the sponsor of the clinical trial. The contract holds all parties who sign it accountable for their performance, and requires that all parties fulfill their obligations as set forth in the contract. For example, if your institution implements the protocol, accrues patients, and collects data and the sponsor refuses compensation as set forth in the agreement, that is a **breach of contract**.

The clinical trial contract specifies that the trial will be conducted under Good Clinical Practice (GCP) guidelines, establishes the payment schedule, and assigns the rights to publish the findings of the research. The contract includes definitions of indemnification and liability as well as noncompete clauses, which prohibit signatories from participating in trials that compete with this study.

■ Contract Negotiation

Negotiating a contract can be a tricky business. If your organization does not have a contracts and grants department or specific legal counsel, hire an attorney, with medical contracts experience, to review the terms of the agreement and to negotiate any changes with the sponsor's legal department.

When reviewing the contract, be clear about what you want covered. Do you want publication rights? Do you want confidentiality and indemnification? The contract should state clearly how the participating institution will be paid by the sponsor. Will payments be made quarterly, after monitoring visits? Be sure that the onus is placed on the sponsor to conduct monitoring visits in a timely fashion. Again, if the sponsor fails to do so, then a penalty must be paid. Whatever you decide about the specific terms, try to keep the contract simple.

■ Signing the Contract

Nothing is worse than being faced with an unsigned contract after weeks and perhaps months of institutional review board (IRB) submissions, organizing the various components of the study, screening potential patients, and being ready to get started. Everything comes to a screeching halt while you wait for the details to be worked out.

Once agreed upon, the principal investigator and the sponsor sign the contract. Some sponsors may agree to have the site initiation while contract negotiations are under way, but generally the study drug is not shipped until the contract has been signed. Occasionally, a sponsor anxious to get a trial going may ship the drug before the contract is signed. To avoid liability and to protect your right to receive payment for services rendered, you must *not* accrue any patients until the contract has been signed.

■ Protocol Amendments

Be aware that a protocol amendment may impact the contract. For example, if the amendment requires DNA or genetic testing, additional blood may need to be drawn. The cost of the additional testing may prompt a budget revision, which in turn may prompt a contract revision. Also, any change that involves new technology may impact liability and will likely necessitate a contract change. If revised, the contract must again be reviewed by legal counsel and signed again by the principal investigator and the sponsor. Do not proceed with any new procedures until a revised consent and protocol have IRB approval and the revised contract has been signed.

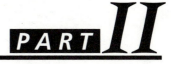

PART II

Setting the Foundation

- *Initiating the Protocol*
- *Preparing for Treatment*

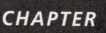
Initiating the Protocol

After approval is received from the institutional review board (IRB), the budget is agreed to, and the contract is signed, it is time for the site initiation visit. The sponsor is mandated by the FDA to visit sites involved in the study to ensure everything is in order.

■ Investigators' Meeting

Initiations can be done a variety of ways. If the protocol is large (usually phase III) and has multiple sites, the sponsor may host an investigators' meeting. These meetings usually take place over a couple of days at a nice hotel in some fun city. On the first day, the protocol is reviewed with investigators and study coordinators. On the second day, the case report forms used for data collection are reviewed.

Become well acquainted with a protocol prior to attending an investigators' meeting, as it will be an opportunity for you to ask questions such as exactly how the information should be reported. The other thing to remember is *have fun!* Pharmaceutical companies expend a great effort to entertain you during this weekend. *ENJOY!*

■ Site Visit

The sponsor or the **contract research organization** (CRO) that the sponsor has hired to monitor the protocol or both must conduct a site visit at your institution. During the site visit, they will meet with the investigational drug pharmacist to inspect where the drug will be stored and to review the pharmacy dispensing log to assure that accurate drug accountability records will be kept. The dispensing pharmacy, the clinic, and the treatment area where the patients will be treated will also be visited.

■ Site Initiation Visit

On occasion, the site visit is combined with the site initiation visit, which can vary in length from a half day with the study monitor, sometimes called clinical research associate (CRA), to a full day with several representatives of the sponsor and CRO. The site initiation visit usually includes a formal presentation by the sponsor's medical monitor, describing the science behind the study and discussing results of the preclinical data. Such presentations can be fairly technical but usually are quite interesting. The presentation should be attended by as many of the departments involved in executing the protocol as possible—for example, representatives from the pharmacy and lab, treatment room manager and/or nurses, the principal investigator, and the subinvestigators should all attend. After the protocol is presented, the study monitor, coordinator, and data manager review the case report forms.

■ Case Report Forms

The sponsor provides case report forms (CRFS) to facilitate collection of the data. The forms are placed in large notebooks that are generally divided into several sections: inclusion/exclusion criteria, screening, cycles, end of study, follow-up, concomitant medications, adverse events, and serious adverse events. Be sure to review the CRFs when you receive them to ensure that the data asked for is consistent with the requirements of the protocol. Careful comparison of these documents is critical to identify any data being requested on the forms that either is not specified in the protocol or that you may have missed in spite of the hundreds of hours you have spent reading the protocol. This will prove helpful when you prepare standardized chemotherapy orders for the study. (See Chapter 7.)

The best way to review a CRF is to record responses for a hypothetical patient. Until you gain experience, just looking at the pages may not help you to anticipate problems. Be aware that no matter how well you think you understand a protocol, more questions are bound to arise when you begin seeing patients and recording data.

Preparing for Treatment

To date, you have secured institutional review board (IRB) approval, an approved budget, and a signed contract; your site initiation has taken place; your case report forms (CRFs) have arrived; and the drug has been shipped. Be aware that some pharmacies require as much as 48 hours after receipt of the drug before the first patient can be treated. It may take that long for the pharmacy to inventory the drug, place it on the shelf under the proper storage conditions, and disperse it to the dispensing pharmacy for preparation for patient use. It is always wise to alert the pharmacy that a study drug is being shipped and notify the pharmacy as to when you expect to treat your first patient. Failure to do so can result in long delays in actually treating the patient and leaves lots of people very unhappy, especially you.

■ Preparing the Orders

Once you have a clear understanding of the treatment and the data collection requirements, begin writing the **standardized chemotherapy orders** (Figure 7–1). The orders should identify the protocol with a simplified name, IRB number, the patient's study number, diagnosis, height, weight, the patient's body surface area (BSA), and allergies.

Chemotherapy Order

Date	**A Phase I Study of ABC123 Given Twice Weekly for 4 Weeks Followed by a 2-Week Rest**
	IRB# 99-09-71
	Principal Investigator: Find A. Cure, MD Study Coordinator: Inta Detail, RN
	Co-Investigators: James Script, MD, Meda Cine, MD, Proto Kol, MD
	Patient # _____ Diagnosis: _____ Cycle: __1__, Week __1__
	Height: _____ cm Weight: _____ kg BSA: _____
	Allergies: _____
1.	Please draw CBC, Chemistry, and PT, PTT, and run the CBC STAT.
2.	See Worksheet on back for Vital Signs and PK Sampling
3.	If Hemoglobin >9, Platelets >100,000, and ANC >1.5, then
4.	**ABC123 200 mg/m² = _____ mg IV @150 mL/hour**
	Start Time: _____ Stop Time: _____ Volume: _____
	All PKs have been drawn, spun, and frozen according to protocol.
	Treating RN Signature: _____
	MD Signature

(FRONT)

Figure 7–1 Sample standardized chemotherapy orders. (IRB = institutional review board; BSA = body surface area; PT = prothrombin time; PTT = partial thromboplastin time; PK = pharmacokinetic; ANC = absolute neutrophil count.)

The orders must include all necessary vital signs, any lab parameters needed to ensure safe treatment of the patient, and special instructions for the person administering the treatment. Note that you may need several different orders to accommodate different requirements on the various days of treatments. For example, if the patient is being treated twice weekly but labs are required only once each week, your orders will need to reflect that difference (Figure 7–2).

If your study requires frequent monitoring of vital signs and pharmacokinetic (PK) draws, creating a worksheet on the back of the orders is useful (Figure 7–3). Placing all of that information on the order sheet itself makes the page complicated visually and can result in omissions of data by the treating nurse. A worksheet helps the treating nurse to see what the requirements are at specific times and to record the data clearly. Note also the statement about PKs on the chemotherapy order (see Figure 7–1):

All PKs have been drawn, spun, and frozen according to protocol.

Many monitors and auditors require proof that the PKs are drawn and handled according to the protocol; this statement provides such a record.

If the drug will be administered in a treatment area, it is wise to give a copy of the orders to the head nurse for review before they are finalized. An objective review by one not familiar with the protocol often yields helpful suggestions.

■ Laboratory Requisitions

Prepare standardized laboratory requisitions for the blood tests that will be required on the various treatment days. Just like the orders, you may need to prepare different requisitions for different days.

Depending on the institution's billing system, you also will likely need to write separate requisitions for tests that will be billed to insurance and for the tests that will be billed to the sponsor, these latter costs are included in the budget. Including the words DO *NOT* BILL TO PATIENT and the study account number on the requisition is sometimes helpful.

Before you begin the requisition process, find out what your laboratory and financial people prefer. Billing errors are time-consuming and avoidable.

Chemotherapy Order

Date	A Phase I Study of ABC123 Given Twice Weekly for 4 Weeks Followed by a 2-Week Rest
	IRB# 99-09-71
	Principal Investigator: Find A. Cure, MD Study Coordinator: Inta Detail, RN
	Co-Investigators: James Script, MD, Meda Cine, MD, Proto Kol, MD
	Patient # _____ Diagnosis: _____ Cycle: __1__, Day __4__
	Height: _____ cm Weight: _____ kg BSA: _____
	Allergies: _____
1.	Preinfusion Vital Signs: BP _____/_____ HR _____ R _____ T _____
2.	**ABC123 200 mg/m² = _____ mg IV @150 mL/hour**
	Start Time: _____ Stop Time: _____ Volume: _____
3.	Postinfusion Vital Signs: BP _____/_____ HR _____ R _____ T _____
	Treating RN Signature: _____
	MD Signature

(BACK)

Figure 7–2 Sample standardized chemotherapy orders (IRB = institutional review board; BSA = body surface area; BP = blood pressure; HR = heart rate; R = respiration; T = temperature; ANC = absolute neutrophil count)

Worksheet
Cycle 1, Day 1

Time Point	Scheduled Time	Actual Time	Vital Signs				PK Sampling
Preinfusion			BP ___/___	HR ___	R ___	T ___	Green-top tube*
30 minutes after start			BP ___/___	HR ___	R ___	T ___	Green-top tube*
Immediately postinfusion			BP ___/___	HR ___	R ___	T ___	Green-top tube*
30 minutes after stop			BP ___/___	HR ___	R ___	T ___	Green-top tube*
60 minutes after stop			BP ___/___	HR ___	R ___	T ___	Green-top tube*
90 minutes after stop			XXXXXXXXXXXXXXXXXXXXXXXXXXXXXXXX				Green-top tube*
120 minutes after stop			BP ___/___	HR ___	R ___	T ___	Green-top tube*
150 minutes after stop			XXXXXXXXXXXXXXXXXXXXXXXXXXXXXXXX				Green-top tube*
180 minutes after stop			BP ___/___	HR ___	R ___	T ___	Green-top tube*

*Please place green-top tubes immediately on ice. Spin at 3,500 rpm for 10 minutes in cold centrifuge and freeze at −20°C.

Figure 7–3 Worksheet on back of standardized chemotherapy order (BP = blood pressure; HR = heart rate; R = respiration; T = temperature)

■ Study Packets

To avoid unnecessary haste and omissions when the patient screening process begins, prepare study packets for the protocol. The screening packet should include a copy of the consent form, lab slips premarked for the required lab tests, and requisitions for EKG, CT scans, and chest x-rays as required in the screening procedures for the protocol. If the study requires a registration form or a screening checklist include it as part of the screening packet. Also, be sure to include an appointment form so that the patient can schedule the appropriate appointments for treatment (see below).

You might also choose to prepare cycle packets that include all of the chemotherapy orders, laboratory requisitions, EKG requisitions, and other documents needed for each cycle of the study. By compiling required documentation ahead of time, you will avoid significant errors of omission and the stress of last-minute work.

■ Appointment Scheduling

Patients receive so much information when enrolling in a clinical trial that sometimes the most important information—when to show up—gets lost. Give the patient as much information as possible in writing. Setting up appointment scheduling forms (Figure 7–4) by cycle, if cycle requirements differ, will help keep confusion and telephone calls to a minimum.

Add important patient instructions to the appointment scheduling form, particularly if a study has many confusing requirements. Fill in the dates on which the patient must be seen, and then send the patient to the appointment desk with the form. The form tells the scheduler how much time the treatment room staff needs for each visit. When all of the times are filled in, make a copy of the form and keep it in the patient's research chart (to be discussed in Chapter 9) so that you too will know when the patient is coming.

■ Inservicing the Treatment Staff

Shortly before you plan to treat the first patient, set up an inservice for the treatment room staff. Invite the pharmacist, the lab manager, and anyone else who may be involved in executing the protocol. Prepare a handout with information about the study drug and its administration.

Briefly discuss the preclinical data pertaining to possible side effects.

ABC123
Patient Appointments
CYCLE 1

Patient Name: _____ **ID #** _____

Day	Date	Time	Comments	Notes
1			ABC123 4-hour visit for PKs	Fast after midnight prior to appointment
2			Nonfasting blood test	Okay to eat before appointment
8			ABC123 4-hour visit for PKs	Fast after midnight; bring diary
15			ABC123 Nonfasting blood test Appt with RN	Bring diary
22			Nonfasting blood test	
29	XXXXXXXXX	XXXXXXXXX	Rest week	
36			Cycle 1 assessment Appt with MD	

All PKs to be drawn ☐ peripherally or ☐ via portacath

Figure 7–4 Sample appointment scheduling form (PK = pharmacokinetic)

Spend more time reviewing administration issues. For example, what is the route of administration, the length of time of infusion, are premedications required, and is the drug a known vesicant?

The dispensing pharmacist will have received detailed instructions about preparing the drug for administration from the sponsor. Ask the lab manager to review the lab requisitions.

Attach a copy of the treatment orders so that the nurses can become familiar with them and ask questions if there is something that is unclear. You may even change the orders based on their input. If PK sampling is required, review the importance of exact timing and proper handling of the specimens. Remind them to page you if any unexpected side effects are seen during the treatment and give them plenty of time to ask questions.

Let everyone know that their role is important to the safe treatment of the patients and the success of the study. Bringing food (bagels or cookies) is always appreciated and serves as an upfront thank you for their hard work, past and future.

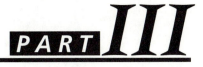

PART III

The Clinical Side

- *The Enrollment Process*
- *Treating the Patient*
- *Pharmacokinetic Sampling*

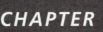

The Enrollment Process

■ Enrolling Patients

Potential candidates for clinical trials are identified in several ways. If an institution is large and provides primary care to patients, it probably has many candidates for phase II and phase III trials. At a major academic medical center that serves as a tertiary facility, the vast majority of patients will be referred by primary oncologists who seek the faculty's expertise in determining the best treatment options. Such patients are likely candidates for phase I studies and perhaps some phase II trials. Potential patients may be identified by the principal investigator, a coinvestigator, other physicians both within and outside the participating institution, nurses, family members, and the patients themselves.

Today, many patients are well-informed consumers. Patients or their advocates who are seeking treatment read articles, listen to talk shows, and surf the Internet. However, in some centers, or for some trials with narrow inclusion criteria, however, recruitment may be difficult. In such cases, you must be creative and resourceful when recruiting patients. For example, if you were running a trial in untreated colorectal cancer, you might contact the gastroenterologists and gastrointestinal surgeons in your institution and in the surrounding community to let them know about the study; these physicians often diagnose the disease and make the first referral for treatment. Be sure that people within your institution are aware of planned and ongoing clinical trials.

You might also check the Internet to locate local chapters of national alliances and to identify local support groups. Providing an information sheet (see Chapter 2) to these organizations may help to recruit patients.

Important Note

If you plan to advertise or publicize a study in an effort to recruit patients, the copy must first be seen and approved by the institutional review board (IRB).

And speaking of the Internet, why not start a Web site for your research program? You can put information about who to call for information and a map on how to reach your facility. You can also have information about each of your trials with inclusion/exclusion criteria (simplified) and a brief description of the trial. You'd be amazed at how many people surf the Internet looking for information about potential treatments.

■ Screening by Telephone

The screening process often begins with a telephone call. If a receptionist or new patient appointment desk serves as the first point of contact with a prospective patient, you might want to create a form that will help clarify whether the person may be appropriate for a clinical trial (Figure 8–1).

Even if a patient is referred by another physician, it is strongly recommended that contact be made with that patient by phone before he or she visits the clinic. Carefully review the patient's history, performance status, and current medications to determine eligibility. Ask open-ended questions. Compare "How do you spend your day?" with "Are you out of bed more than 50 percent of the day?" Which question do you think will generate a more accurate account of the patient's performance status?

Although many patients will tell you that they had no medical problems prior to their cancer diagnosis, close review of their medications might reveal an antihypertensive or a cholesterol-lowering medication. If the patient mentions a medication with which you are

New Patient Screening Sheet

Date _____   Screened by _____

PATIENT INFORMATION

Patient Name _____

DOB _____   SS # _____

Day Phone # _____   Home Phone # _____

Address _____

Referred by _____   Phone # _____

Diagnosis _____   Date Diagnosed _____

Metastatic to   Bone   Brain   Liver   Lung   Lymph Node   Other

Surgery _____

Chemotherapy/Drugs	Date Started	Date Completed
1. _____	_____	_____
2. _____	_____	_____
3. _____	_____	_____
4. _____	_____	_____

Radiation	Date Started	Date Completed
1. _____	_____	_____
2. _____	_____	_____

INSURANCE INFORMATION _____
_____
_____

COMMENTS _____

Figure 8–1 New patient screening sheet

unfamiliar, look it up. The drug, or the condition it treats, might be grounds for an exclusion from the protocol.

Explain the protocol to the patient, being sure to discuss the study procedures and frequency of visits. If possible, fax a copy of the consent form to the patient, or if time allows, mail it. Patients can then read the consent form and share it with their families in a comfortable environment, free from the stress of a busy clinic. Invite the patient to call you, after reading the consent form, with any questions.

Do not schedule a patient for a screening visit until all issues surrounding insurance, commitment to study procedures, housing, and transportation have been discussed. If there is any doubt in your mind about the patient's qualifications or commitment to the study, be sure to schedule the screening visit well in advance of the patient's expected enrollment date. This is particularly important if a patient is scheduled to fill an opening in a phase I study, where each succeeding cohort is dependent on the previous cohort completing a cycle. Failure to enroll a patient in a timely manner in a phase I study will delay the enrollment of all subsequent patients and cohorts.

> ### Important Note
>
> It is better to delay a week to complete appropriate screening tests and to be sure of a patient's eligibility than to rush an ineligible patient into study.

Request that the patient bring to the screening visit copies of a recent medical history and physical exam; reports of the most recent CT scans and bone scans, if appropriate; the most recent labs; previous treatment history including surgery, chemotherapy and radiation; and the report of the original pathology. Do *not* take responsibility for collecting such data yourself. A patient's willingness to gather this information and to supply it when requested may be a good indication of their early commitment to the study. It is preferable to have the patient simply bring the records to clinic at the time of the appointment to avoid a variety of pitfalls that result in inadequate or missing information to clearly determine eligibility.

> ### Reminder
>
> Patient confidentiality is an inherent part of the medical profession. Remind staff members that a breach of confidentiality is unacceptable and is grounds for dismissal.

■ Preparing a Research Chart

Many research centers find it helpful to set up a special chart that includes all records pertinent to a patient's participation in a specific clinical trial. Research charts, often called *shadow charts* or *dummy charts*, are kept in the research office and contain copies of the patient's records. All original documents *must* be kept in the patient's medical record at your institution.

The research chart should be divided into sections, such as progress notes, lab results, radiology reports, other studies (for example, EKGs, ultrasound studies, etc.) pathology reports, previous treatment, and miscellaneous. In a large medical facility, the patient's medical record is not always available when the patient is being seen in clinic. Also, trying to locate the latest lab or CT results in the medical record may be next to impossible due to delays in filing or to the sheer volume of pages.

Understand that a research chart is *not* a source document. The original medical record always serves as source documentation to verify information. A research chart, though it may require some time to keep current, is well worth the effort.

■ The Screening Visit

Well, the big day has finally arrived and you will soon start to see patients for enrollment in the study. If the patient's information has been received in advance, be sure to review it, and place it in the research chart, under the previous treatment section. Highlighting all significant information will help define the salient points for the physician and save time in clinic.

The Waiting Room

Try to meet the patient in the waiting room, introduce yourself, and give the patient a copy of the consent form if it was not sent earlier. If the consent has recently been revised, be sure that the patient has the most current version. While waiting, the patient has time to read the consent and prepare questions prior to seeing the physician.

Medical Records

If the patient has brought copies of his or her records as requested, retrieve them at this time and begin to review them. If the patient has failed to bring the records as requested, or if the records have been faxed to nobody knows who, now is the time to find out. Call the referring physician's office and request that the records be refaxed or that they identify where the records were sent *before* the patient is placed in an examination room. Once received, organize the records into sections following the research chart format and then arrange each section in chronological order. As a rule, the most recent labs and CTs are the only ones needed. Some patients will bring every lab drawn since their diagnosis. Many records come with multiple copies of the same information but some important piece of information is missing. Organizing and reviewing the records up front saves time and helps the physician.

Vital Signs and Other Essentials

When the patient is placed in the examination room, be sure that someone has taken the patient's vital signs *and* height and weight. Nothing is worse than being ready to treat a patient, only to discover that the height needed to calculate the BSA is missing.

Medications, Allergies, and Pregnancy

During the screening visit, inquire about the patient's current medications, including dose, frequency, and indication for use. You might also need to find out *when* the patient started taking that medication. Most studies require that you record all medications taken within 4 to 6 weeks of enrollment. Therefore, be sure to ask the patient whether he or she was taking a medication but stopped within the last month or so. Remember that blood transfusions are considered medication. Also, discuss the patient's allergies and identify the reaction experienced.

The physician *must* address contraceptive counseling in the interview and in the consultation note. If the patient is female, have a frank discussion about her ability to become pregnant. If she is under 55 years old and has not been surgically sterilized, request a pregnancy test. Even if her partner has had a vasectomy, request a pregnancy test. Advise the patient that a pregnancy test is being ordered because of unknown, but potential, side effects to an unborn child. The protocol will state if a serum pregnancy test is needed or a urine pregnancy is acceptable.

Other Options and Informed Consent

Be sure that the principal investigator has discussed all of the patient's treatment options. In cancer clinical trials these include: best supportive care (treatment for symptoms only); standard, FDA-approved drugs; or experimental therapy. Particularly in phase I studies, patients have high expectations regarding the success of the therapy and may discount potential toxicities.[1] As part of the consenting process, patients must be told of all known side effects and also that there may be side effects that are not yet known, even death.

Some patients may want to sign the consent without reading it. Do *not* allow this. No matter how anxious the patient may be, signing an unread consent is dangerous business.

After reading the consent, some patients may become frightened or worried about the possible side effects of the experimental therapy. Reassure patients with what you currently know about the drug, but do not be overconfident. Reiterate that there are no guarantees. Choosing to enroll in a clinical trial is a decision that the patient must make of his or her own free will. Beware of patients with overzealous families. Again, you must be certain that the patient wants to participate in the study; a patient should not participate just to please the family.

Signing and Distributing the Consent

If it is determined that the patient is appropriate for participation in the study and has been fully informed, the patient then signs the consent.

Important Note

Recall that the patient must sign the consent *before* any study-related tests or procedures can be done.

The FDA is very particular about that. The patient must also date the consent. Adding the time signed to the consent will help clarify the fact that the patient was consented prior to blood work or any other study procedures if they are being done on the same day as the screening visit.

Who must sign the consent varies from institution to institution. In all cases, the patient's signature attests to the fact that he or she has read, understands, and agrees to the terms of the consent. Generally, the person who performs the consenting process must also sign the consent.

If English is not the patient's primary language, the person acting as translator also must sign the consent, and it should be written in the progress note that a translator was present and explained the consent to the patient. It is preferable that the translator not be a family member of the patient. In some cultures, the elderly are spared the bad news. If you do not understand what the patient is being told, you cannot attest to the fact that the patient has been fully informed. Remember that the copy of the consent given to the patient must be in his or her primary language.

After all signatures are obtained, make several copies of the consent.

Give one copy to the patient and place one copy in the research chart. (The screening visit note should state that the patient was given an opportunity to ask questions, which were answered, and that a copy of the consent was given to the patient.) In some institutions, the original consent is placed in the patient's medical record; in others, the original consents are kept in one place for a specific trial. If the latter is the case at your facility, place a copy in the medical record. Be *extremely* careful with the original signed consent. Do not let it out of your possession until you have personally filed it in the appropriate place.

◼ The Investigator's Responsibilities

The physician must review the patient's history and past treatment to satisfy that the patient is indeed eligible for the study. It is also his or her responsibility to explain the trial and its possible side effects to the patient. The physician must also provide contraceptive counseling and answer all of the patient's questions.

Know what information you need the physician to document for the baseline screening. For example, do you need a performance status? What specific body systems need to be addressed in the physical exam? Is a rectal exam required? Don't expect the physician to remember these details; it is the study coordinator's responsibility to be sure the correct data are collected.

If the study is being conducted in a teaching institution, and a fellow, nurse practitioner, or student sees the patient at screening or at any time during the study, a note must be written or dictated by a physician or nurse who is an investigator in the study. Once the patient's clinic visit is concluded with the physician, be sure to make a copy of any outside records that you need and don't let them out of your sight. Often, if outside documents go to a medical records department not fixed to a chart, you can kiss them good-bye and count on hours of atoning for your sin.

◼ Confirming Contacts

Once the physician has completed explaining the study and examining the patient, review the study procedures once again with the patient. The patient needs to be told what tests are required now and where to get them. The patient should also be given the appointment schedule (see Figure 7–3) and be assisted when making the first appointment for treatment.

Be sure you know how to reach the patient in case any of the screening tests need to be repeated or (heaven forbid) to inform the patient that he or she is not eligible. Remember, if a patient is from out of town, the computer will probably only give you the home address and phone number. A phone number in Texas is not useful if you need to reach the patient in Los Angeles this afternoon. Be sure to give the patient your card. Be generous. Give cards to the significant other or anyone else who may be involved in the patient's participation in the study. Tell them if anything comes up prior to the first appointment to call you.

■ Completing the Process

Review *all* of the screening labs carefully. Be sure to order the appropriate tumor marker, if applicable. If you failed to order something you need, or if the lab failed to run everything you requested, you generally have 48 hours to correct the error, provided that the appropriate tubes were drawn. Most labs keep a patient's serum sample for that time period; after 48 hours, the serum no longer gives accurate results.

Do not make the mistake of examining just the test results required by the inclusion/exclusion criteria and miss the fact that a patient is hypercalcemic or hypokalemic. If you find a lab abnormality at screening, discuss it with the investigator. If it is significant, the patient may need immediate treatment. If the value seems unlikely to be accurate, repeat the test. Lab errors can happen. If the abnormality is insignificant, the investigator may decide to ask the sponsor for an exception to enroll the patient.

As soon as the decision is made to ask for an exception, e-mail the request to the physician in charge of the study, the sponsor's medical monitor. For example, you may know before the screening appointment that the study candidate had a CT scan 2 weeks ago which will be 4 days past the protocol's date requirement. Or, you may find during a phone conversation that the candidate's last dose of chemotherapy will be 3 weeks and 6 days before starting the study drug, 1 day short of the date requirement. Explain the condition that requires the exception specifying the exact section of the protocol that is not met by the candidate. If the medical monitor has any concerns or questions, they can be addressed prior to proceeding with more screening procedures.

Complete the sponsor's registration form, and fax it to the sponsor as soon as possible. If you have asked for an exception for a patient to be enrolled, be sure that information is noted on the registration form as well as in the medical record. Be sure that the registration is signed and returned by the sponsor *before* the patient is treated. Remember to take time-zone differences into account.

If an exception has been granted, the sponsor should send an exception letter along with the registration form. If you have not received an exception letter, then pursue it. Use e-mail to document any discussion with the sponsor about exceptions. Send the e-mail to the monitor and print a hard copy for the file. Exceptions that are granted but not documented will haunt you during the monitoring process.

Place the original exception letter in the regulatory binder under correspondence. Place copies of the exception letter in the patient's medical record, research chart, and CRf to facilitate verification of the exception when the monitor reviews the record.

Most IRBs require notification of exceptions. Check with your IRB for its preference, but for most exceptions (for example, a CT a few days out of window, a platelet count of 95,000 rather than 100,000) a monthly report to the IRB will suffice. Some IRBs may simply request that exception information be placed in the annual report when the study is renewed. If this is the case, one copy of the report should be placed in the regulatory binder.

■ Reference

1. Chang, J. D., Hitt, J., Koczwara, B., Schulman, K. A., Burnett, C. B., Gaskin, D. J., Rowland, J. H., & Meropol, N. J. (2000). Impact of quality of life on patient expectations regarding phase I clinical trials. *Journal of Clinical oncology, 18* (2), 421–428.

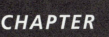

CHAPTER 9

Treating the Patient

■ The Orders

Can you believe it; you are actually going to treat a patient! Finally! At some institutions, you may be asked to calculate the body surface area (BSA) and the dose. If that is the case, the physician must recalculate and confirm both the BSA and dose. More typically, though, you will present the uncompleted orders to the physician and will be responsible for ensuring that the orders are completed and signed well before they are needed in the treatment unit. Remember that a physician who is an investigator in the study must *always* sign the orders.

A copy of the **signed orders and a copy of the signature page of the consent form** must then be sent to the dispensing pharmacy. If more than one pharmacy is used during the treatment (for example, outpatient and inpatient), each pharmacy must receive a copy of the consent.

> ### *Time-Saving Hint*
>
> Prepare all orders and lab requisitions for the entire cycle at one time. This approach will avoid mistakes and eliminates running around for signatures at the last minute.

It is best to maintain the orders and laboratory requisitions in the research office until the day prior to the patient's scheduled visit. That way, if changes to the dosage, premedications, or lab tests are required, the orders are accessible. Keeping the orders close by is also the best way to prevent things from being misplaced.

Place the signed orders and labs in a **tickler file**, which is a file ordered chronologically. Move the orders and labs to the appropriate area the night before the patient is due. Make a habit of reviewing the orders in the tickler file each day or each week, *before* they are sent to the treatment area, to make sure that all patients scheduled to be treated have orders and that the orders are correct and up-to-date.

■ Recording the Patient's Visits

Some protocols require that the physician see the patient prior to each treatment, and others require that the patient be seen only once a month. Regardless, the study coordinator/data manager should see the patient each time the patient is scheduled for a visit, at least during the first cycle.

Prepare a progress note for the patient prior to each visit (Figure 9–1). The progress note should include the patient's name, medical record number, diagnosis, previous performance status (ECOG or KPS), date of last tumor marker and restaging scans, date of next tumor marker and restaging scans, and all current adverse events. You will notice that in the sample progress note in Figure 9–1, a signature is required in each section. Each person who records information on the progress note must identify his or her entries with a signature. For example, if the clinic staff records the vital signs, you record the adverse events and conduct the review of systems (that is, the patient's subjective symptoms), and the investigator performs the physical exam, all three parties must sign the progress note.

> ### *Reminder*
>
> If you work at a major medical center, a forms committee most likely reviews and approves all new forms that are developed. Any unapproved forms contained in the medical record are often removed when the record reaches the medical record department. Therefore, when creating a progress note, begin with your institution's standard form and make modifications to it.

Multidisciplinary Progress Note

TRIAL: _____   Cycle: _____   Week: _____

Vital Signs:	Allergies:	WBC: ____ ANC: ____
Weight:		Hgb: _____
Height:	Medications:	Platelets: _____
BP:		Prior ECOG: _____
HR:		Today's ECOG _____
R:		Last CT Date: _____
T:		Next CT Due: _____
BSA:		Tumor Marker: _____ Value: _____ on ___/___/___
Signature:		Prior Tumor Marker Value: _____ on ___/___/___

_____ year old   M   F   with _____(diagnosis)

Adverse Events	Start Date	Stop Date	Grade	Relation to Study Drug
				Signature

REVIEW OF SYSTEMS:

EXAM:
Appearance:
HEENT:
Chest:
CV:
Abdomen:
Extremities:
Neurological:
Skin:
Musculoskeletal:
Assessment:
Plan:
MD Signature

Figure 9–1 Sample progress note (BP = blood pressure; HR = heart rate; R = respiration; T = temperature; BSA = body surface area; ANC = absolute neutrophil count; Hgb = hemoglobin; ECOG = performance status; HEENT = head, eyes, ears, nose, throat; CV = cardiovascular)

During a patient visit, review any side effects the patient may be experiencing. Listen carefully to what the patient describes and determine whether the symptom was present at baseline or whether it is different from the baseline symptoms. If so, record it as an adverse event (AE). If you suspect that the symptom is significant, discuss it with the physician. Even if you are certain that the study drug did not cause the symptom, you must still record it. Any laboratory abnormality must also be recorded as an AE, unless the investigator finds it not to be clinically significant. Check the **toxicity criteria** attached to the protocol to determine the grade of the AE. The toxicity table gives objective data to determine the grade of the AE.

Also record on the progress note any changes in the patient's medications. If a medication was stopped, record the stop date. If a new medication was started, record the start date. If a patient starts a new medication, it is likely that he or she has had an adverse event that required treatment. For example, if a patient received lorazepam (Ativan) for nausea during the infusion, you will need to note the lorazepam as a concomitant medication and the nausea as an AE. (See Chapter 11 for more on data collection requirements.)

■ Cycle Assessments

Generally, at the end of every cycle, the patient is required to have a reassessment visit. These end-of-cycle visits usually include physical examination with assessment of palpable masses, as well as urinalysis, lab work, and EKG. At each cycle assessment, all of the patient's current medications should be reviewed as a doublecheck that nothing has been missed during the preceding weeks. If a tumor marker is being followed, it should be drawn at this visit. Prepare a progress note (see Figure 9–1) for this visit, and ensure that all vital signs and details of the physical examination are recorded. Copy the progress note for the research chart, and place the original in the patient's medical record.

■ Restaging

A clinical trial specifies restaging of patients at prescribed intervals to assess response to the study treatment. Restaging consists of repeating the same radiographic studies that were done at baseline and comparing the new results with the earlier studies. A patient's response can be complicated to assess because of many clinical variances: What if a patient has clinical benefit, less pain, but the CT scan shows an increase in the size of the tumors, progressive disease? Is the specified time period, for example 6 weeks, long enough for the patient to have a response? Would treating the patient for 12 weeks before restaging yield different, more positive, results? Nonetheless, the time frame and the method of determining response must be standardized in a clinical trial.

The Southwest Oncology Group (SWOG) Response Criteria (1999) has defined *measurable disease* as bidimensionally measurable lesions with clearly defined margins by (1) medical photography (skin or oral lesions) or plain x-ray, with at least one diameter 0.5 centimeters or greater (bone lesions not included), or (2) CT, MRI, or other imaging study, or (3) palpation, with both diameters 2 centimeters or greater.[1] For patients with measurable disease, most existing studies define the criteria for response as (1) complete response, (2) partial response, (3) stable disease, and (4) progressive disease.

Complete Response

Complete response is defined as the total disappearance of all measurable and evaluable clinical evidence of cancer, observed on at least two assessments that were at least 4 weeks apart. The patients must also exhibit no increase in cancer-associated symptomatology and no decrease in performance status due to the disease.

Partial Response

A *partial response* constitutes at least a 50 percent reduction in the size of all measurable tumor areas, as determined by the sum of the products of the greatest length and the maximum width of all measurable lesions. No lesion may progress and no new lesion may appear. The partial response parameters must have been present for at least two assessments that were at least 4 weeks apart. A 25 to 50 percent reduction in the size of all measurable tumor areas, with no evidence of new lesion(s), that has been present for at least two assessments that were at least 4 weeks apart would qualify as a *minor response.*

For those who are followed for tumor response by tumor markers only, a 75 percent reduction from baseline value, measured on two consecutive dates that were at least 4 weeks apart, qualifies as a minor response.

Stable Disease

Stable disease exists when a patient fails to qualify for either a response or progressive disease.

Progressive Disease

Progressive disease is defined as an increase of 25 percent or more in the size of all measurable tumor areas, as measured by the sum of the products of the greatest length and maximum width, or the appearance of any new lesion(s).

Even though new CT scans are compared with the most recent studies, the total tumor burden of the current studies must be compared to the original baseline studies to determine whether there has been progression or response since starting the study drug. If the disease is measurable, this comparison is done by mathematical calculation. The radiologist *must* compare the same lesions from each study for accurate response determination. As you can see, the criteria is well-defined and does not allow for the clinical variances mentioned earlier. For example, a patient with improvement in pain but 26 percent growth will be taken off the study for progressive disease. At the same time, the patient with 24 percent growth but increased pain stays in the study because the criteria says the disease is stable.

If the lesions are not discrete enough to yield exact measurements, the disease will be considered **evaluable** only, rather than measurable. *Evaluable disease* has been defined by the SWOG Response Criteria as unidimensionally measurable lesions, masses with margins not clearly defined, lesions with both diameters less than 0.5 diameters, lesions on scan with either diameter smaller than the distance between cuts, palpable lesions with either diameter less than 2 centimeters, or bone disease. Tumor markers which have been shown to be highly correlated with extent of disease are also considered evaluable. Pleural effusions, ascites or disease that is only documented by indirect evidence, such as lab values, is considered *non-evaluable.*[1]

Clearly, the assessment of growth or regression may be subjective, and the investigator must make the response determination. Be sure that the investigator clearly documents the rationale behind the decision.

In an effort to better define responses, SWOG has developed new criteria called Response Evaluation Criteria in Solid Tumors (RECIST). The system provides for a combination assessment of all existing lesions, characterized by target lesions which are measured, and non-target lesions, to extrapolate an overall response to treatment. Target lesions will be selected on the basis of their size (lesions with the longest diameter (LD)) and their suitability for accurate repetitive measurements (either by imaging techniques or clinically). A sum of the LD for all target lesions will be calculated and reported as the baseline sum LD. The baseline sum LD will be used as reference to further characterize the objective tumor response of the measurable dimension of the disease. All other lesions (or sites of disease) will be identified as non-target lesions and will also be recorded as baseline. Measurements will not be required and these lesions will be followed as present or absent.[2] This response criteria is now being identified in many new protocols to determine response.

Study Coordinator's Role

Regardless of the criteria used, the study coordinator has two major responsibilities during restaging:

1. Ensure that all prior CT films are available for the radiologist to read. If the original study was done at another facility, confirm that copies of the films have been received by the radiology department.
2. Ensure that the scans are completed well in advance so that the results are available for the assessment appointment.

If it is determined that the radiographic studies show progressive disease either by growth of the tumor burden by more than the specified percent or the appearance of a new lesion, the patient is terminated from the study. However, if a response or stable disease is seen, the patient continues in the study and will be restaged again at the next prescribed interval.

■ End of Treatment

A patient's participation in a study may be terminated for several reasons. The end point of the study is defined within the protocol. In oncology studies, most frequently the determinant is progressive disease. Alternatively, an AE may result in the patient's removal from the study. Occasionally, patients withdraw consent because they tire of the rigors of the trial, the side effects, or because they want to pursue another therapy. Whatever the reason, it should be documented clearly in the physician's progress note and the plan should read *off study.*

■ Follow-up

Within the first 30 days off study, any patient hospitalizations or death must be reported to the sponsor as a serious adverse event (SAE). Most studies require that the patient be seen approximately 30 days after last receiving the study drug, with the goal of resolving any outstanding AEs that may have been related to the study drug. If such an AE is still present at the follow-up visit, then the patient will be followed until resolution of that event. If a patient will not or cannot return to the facility for a follow-up visit, every effort should be made to obtain a physical examination report and lab results from the physician who is caring for the patient.

As long as the trial remains open, most studies require periodic phone inquiries to determine the patient's disease status and any additional treatment, if applicable. A progress note should be written as a source document for the phone calls. If a patient expires after the 30-day follow-up period, a death report must be filed with the sponsor. After the initial 30 days, a patient's death is *not* classified as an SAE but will require a death report to be filed with the sponsor.

■ References

1. *Southwest Oncology Group Clinical Research Manual.* (1999). Vol. I, Chapters 7-2-7-11.
2. Therasse, P., Arbuck, S. G., Eisenhauer, E. A., Wanders, J., Kaplan, R. S., Rubenstein, L., et al. (2000). New guidelines to evaluate the response to treatment in solid tumors. *Journal of the National Cancer Institute* 92(3), 205–216.

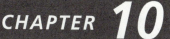
Pharmacokinetic Sampling

■ Understanding Pharmacokinetics

In order to understand how a drug is metabolized, sponsors often require pharmacokinetic (PK) sampling on specific days of a study. These samples are analyzed at special laboratories to determine the drug's metabolites and how long the drug remains in a patient's blood serum. This information is essential to define the drug's mechanism of action and how frequently it may safely be administered. For example, if a drug remains active for only 3 hours, it may need to be administered daily or several times weekly. On the other hand, if a drug remains active for 30 hours, it may safely be administered only weekly or every other week. Drawing PK samples on different treatment days determines if the drug accumulates or if it is completely eliminated between doses.

In some drugs, the metabolite(s) are more potent than the parent compound. In the drug Camptosar, which is approved for the treatment of colon cancer, the active metabolite is SN38; SN38 is 800 to 1,000 times more potent than irinotecan hydrochloride (Camptosar).

■ Preparing for PK Sampling

The sponsor provides the participating institution with all supplies needed to perform PK sampling. Generally, blood is drawn into a green-top, heparinized tube and placed immediately on ice. If the tube is not placed on ice, the metabolites are often lost.

The tube is then transferred to a cold centrifuge and spun at settings prescribed by an appendix in the protocol. Once spun, the serum is pipetted off and placed in one or two plastic cryovials. The cryovials are then transferred into a freezer to be maintained at a specified temperature, usually $-20°$ to $-70°C$.

The sponsor usually supplies labels, with the specific time points noted, for the cryovials. The patient's initials, study number, date the serum is drawn, and the exact time of the draw must be recorded on the labels. For example, the protocol may require that PK samples be drawn preinfusion, at 15 and 30 minutes during the infusion, at the end of the infusion, and often at 5, 10, 15, 30, 60, 90, 120, 150, and 180 minutes postinfusion. It is critical that the person drawing the blood complete the appropriate label with the exact time of the blood draw. If you refer back to Figure 7–2, you will notice that the worksheet has spaces for the phlebotomist to write in the scheduled time as well as the actual time of the draw. A difference of just a few minutes, particularly in a drug with a short half-life can completely confound the results. The need for attention to these details cannot be overstated.

As you may have noted, the hypothetical PK schedule given above requires thirteen PKs per patient. Often, this same schedule is repeated on two or three different days during a cycle. Clearly, within a short period of time, you could accumulate large quantities of cryovials in the freezer. Therefore, frequent shipment of the samples to the laboratory designated to run the assays is probably as important to you as it is to the sponsor's clinical pharmacologist. Great care must be exercised in handling the specimens.

■ Shipping PK Samples

Pharmacokinetic samples *must* remain frozen until they reach the specified laboratory. Often, a requisition must be completed for each patient's specimens indicating the patient's initials, study number, and the date and time of each draw. The specimens must then be matched to the information recorded on the case report form (CRF). They are shipped on dry ice by either messenger, if the special laboratory is local, or overnight carrier.

If overnight shipping is needed, there are other points to consider. For example, the samples must be shipped early in the week because many overnight carriers do not deliver on weekends, and the laboratory may be closed. The boxes must be clearly marked as biohazard material; they also require dry ice labels. All of this preparation must

SPECIMEN CONFIRMATION SHEET

Date _____   Study Name _____

Sponsor _____   Study Number _____

From: Marcy Shipper

Clinical Research Center

Fax: 1-800-555-6543

To: Special Laboratory

The following cryovials have been shipped via _____

Patient's Initials and Number _____   # of Cryovials _____

Patient's Initials and Number _____   # of Cryovials _____

Patient's Initials and Number _____   # of Cryovials _____

Patient's Initials and Number _____   # of Cryovials _____

Patient's Initials and Number _____   # of Cryovials _____

Patient's Initials and Number _____   # of Cryovials _____

Please sign below as confirmation that you have received the above specimens, and fax this form back to the Clinical Research Center immediately. Thank you for your cooperation.

Signature _____

Date _____

Figure 10–1 Sample specimen confirmation sheet

be completed before the overnight company arrives at your facility. Generally, biohazard material cannot simply be dropped off at the same place you drop off your Christmas presents.

Always alert the receiving facility that a shipment is en route. The best way to accomplish this is to fax a notification of shipment that requests that the receiving facility sign and return the confirmation sheet when the samples arrive. The confirmation sheet then serves as documentation of the shipping and receipt of the samples. Figure 10–1 is an example of a typical specimen confirmation sheet.

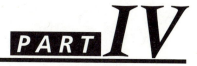

PART IV

The Data Side

- *Data Collection*
- *The Monitoring Process*
- *Closing the Study*

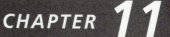
Data Collection

Without a doubt, data collection is the most tedious part of the research process. Even if a center accrues patients rapidly and provides optimal patient care, if data are not reported accurately the validity of the study will be compromised. Remember, no matter how insignificant a detail may seem, the rule of thumb in data collection is *report it*!

■ Understanding the Process

Understanding what happens to the data that you collect and record will help you to provide *clean* data to the sponsor. The information gathered on each patient is recorded on a patient-specific case report form (CRF). Even if you paid close attention to these forms during the site initiation visit, it is likely that you will still have questions when you begin to record data. The sponsor provides a **study reference guide** that explains how to complete the required forms. If the guide fails to answer your questions or if you are uncertain about major data points, speak with the study monitor.

The monitor is responsible for checking the accuracy of data entries. In some studies, the monitor checks *every* entry against source documentation; in others, the monitor spot-checks entries. After the monitor has reviewed and verified the information, the corrections will need to be made either by the study coordinator or the data manager. The original (or top) pages are then removed (or pulled) from the CRF book and sent to the data management company that enters the data into an electronic database. The data is then cross-checked by the computer. If discrepancies or inconsistencies are found, the computer generates queries asking for correction or clarification. Copies of each page of the CRf remain at the site.

■ Screening Data

This section of the CRF documents the patient's past medical history, malignancy history, past treatment history, and results of all baseline labs and radiographic studies. It is strongly recommended that this section be completed by the research nurse or study coordinator. Recording the screening data in this way has two benefits. First, records from outside facilities may not be clear. A study coordinator who understands therapy regimens and can interpret the data is a wise choice for this important function. Second, reviewing and recording patient information allows the coordinator to become familiar with the patient's history, which can only help when evaluating symptoms during the trial.

The patient's concomitant medications are also recorded as part of the screening data. Most sponsors require that the start date and the indication be given for every concomitant medication. This would include any medications that the patient took 4 to 6 weeks prior to entering the study, even if the patient is no longer using those medications. If, after reviewing and recording the screening data, data appears to be missing, make every effort to obtain the needed data well before the monitor's first scheduled visit.

The data manager should review the screening data to become familiar with the patient's profile and review the data entry. Data managers can help retrieve missing data and free the study coordinator for clinical duties.

Past Medical History

Review every detail of the patient's past medical history. Look for consultations, admission histories and physical exams, patient questionnaires, and any progress notes that might help to identify all of the past history. Some monitors require that every fact be recorded, no matter how insignificant it may seem (for example, measles, mumps, rashes, broken fingers). Others will request only significant information. Unless the monitor's wishes were clearly discussed at the site initiation visit, when in doubt, *record it*!

Another sticking point is whether only the diagnosis of a particular problem *or* the diagnosis and all related symptoms must be recorded. For example, if a patient presented with shortness of breath and peripheral edema and was then diagnosed with congestive heart failure, what should be recorded? Most monitors prefer that you *record it all*!

When reviewing a patient's medical history, you may find discrepancies. For example, if one physician incorrectly records something, it is likely that the error will continue to be recorded by every other physician who writes a history for the patient. You may also find inconsistencies in the dates for some procedures.

Helpful Hint

Make a photocopy of the screening pages for use as a worksheet. When all of the data has been clarified, then record it on the CRF. This makes for a much neater document.

Recall that anything a patient experiences right up to the moment of screening is considered past medical history.

Past Treatment History

Patients who have had many past therapies present the greatest challenge to understanding the treatments and their chronology. Few patients bring complete records to the screening visit, so a patient's past treatment history is often the most difficult to record.

Date of Diagnosis

The *date of diagnosis* is defined as the date of the original biopsy. Be sure that you have a copy of the original pathology report on file. Many studies require that a diagnosis be *histologically proven,* which means that tissue was taken from a lesion and determined to be cancer by a pathologist. If the inclusion criteria requires that the diagnosis be histologically proven, you will need to clarify whether patients who were diagnosed by an aspirate only are eligible.

There are also patients for whom only a **presumptive diagnosis** can be made. Depending on the study's inclusion criteria, therefore, such a patient may not be eligible for the study. For example, if a patient presents with an enlarged lymph node in the neck, either a fine-needle aspirate (FNA) or excision of the lymph node is done. If the biopsy is read as metastatic adenocarcinoma, then the patient faces an involved workup to locate the primary site. The workup might include CT scans, bone scans, mammograms, endoscopic examinations, and blood work, including tumor markers. Even if no primary tumor is identified, all of this data helps the oncologist begin formulating treatment decisions. For example, if the tumor marker CA 19.9 is elevated, it is presumed the patient has pancreatic cancer, in spite of the fact that the primary site is really unknown. If the protocol is designed for patients, with pancreatic cancer histologically confirmed the patient is not eligible.

Radiation History

Radiation history should include the exact site radiated, the date on which the radiation treatment began and ended, and the dose. Radiation doses are measured in rads, grays, or centigrays (50 grays = 5,000 centigrays). At the completion of radiation treatment, the radiation oncologist completes a radiation summary, which is the report you need. Occasionally, you may need to request the report from the radiation facility.

Helpful Hint

The patient's informed consent to participate in the study includes the patient's consent to obtain outside records. If you are asked for a release when requesting records, send the pages of the consent that pertain to outside records as well as the signature page.

Chemotherapy History

In order to record the chemotherapy history, first secure a copy of the patient's chemotherapy flow sheets. This section must include all systemic drugs used for the treatment of the cancer, including not only cytotoxic agents, but also hormones (for example, tamoxifen, leuprolide acetate [Lupron]) and drugs used as sensitizers, protectants, or enhancers for the chemotherapy drugs (for example, leucovorin, MESNA). Usually you will need the start and stop dates and the doses as well.

The sponsor may ask how many cycles of a regimen a patient

received and what the response was. Be aware that the patient may have received treatment at several different facilities. When recording a therapy that is experimental write *experimental* after the name of the drug. If the outside records were available at the screening visit, the physician's dictation may help to clarify this information.

Do *not* record any premedications given for chemotherapy, such as antiemetics or dexamethasone (Decadron), because technically they are not part of the chemotherapy regimen. However, if prednisone is given as part of the regimen, it must be recorded. If you are unclear about this distinction, ask the investigator for help.

Baseline Lesion Assessment

Protocols require baseline assessments to determine the extent of a patient's disease at the time of entry into the study. Read the protocol carefully to determine what the window (time line) is for this assessment. Some studies require that the patient have bidimensionally measurable disease; others allow a patient to be followed with evaluable disease or by tumor markers only. For example, many patients with prostate cancer may have only bone lesions that are not bidimensionally measurable. Such patients may be followed by tumor marker—prostate-specific antigen—(PSA) only. Patients with broncheoalveolar carcinoma, a type of non-small-cell lung cancer, may show only thickening of pleural surfaces rather than discrete, measurable masses on CT scan. When you review CRFs at the site initiation visit, check whether the form allows for recording of patients with evaluable disease only. Figure 11–1 is an example of a lesion assessment page that covers all of these possibilities.

Timing

The protocol may require that baseline scans be done within 14 to 28 days prior to starting the study drug. If a patient has had a scan that is outside that window by a matter of days, the sponsor may grant an exception allowing the patient to enter the study without repeating the scans. Remember that insurers will only pay for CT scans every 8 to 12 weeks. Therefore, if a sponsor requires that you repeat a scan 6 weeks after the one scan, bill the sponsor for that scan. *Include such stipulations in your budget.*

Required Studies

Baseline examinations must include all studies necessary to completely define the patient's disease. The patient's known areas of disease as

Lesion Assessment

MEASURABLE LESION(S)

Site	Date Assessed	Method	Measurements
			_____ cm × _____ cm
			_____ cm × _____ cm
			_____ cm × _____ cm

NONMEASURABLE LESION(S)

Site	Date Assessed	Method	Status

STATUS
0 = Not assessed   4 = Decreased
1 = New   5 = Resolved
2 = Increased   6 = Relapsed
3 = Stable   7 = Not applicable

TUMOR MARKER(S)

Marker	Date Assessed	Result	Clinically Significant
			☐ Yes ☐ No
			☐ Yes ☐ No

RESPONSE TO STUDY DRUG
Response determined:
☐ Radiographically   ☐ Tumor Marker   ☐ Other _____

Response: ☐ Complete Response
           ☐ Partial Response   ☐ 25–50% (Minor Response)
                                ☐ >50%
           ☐ Stable Disease
           ☐ Progressive Disease

Figure 11–1 Sample lesion assessment form

well as the diagnosis dictate what studies are performed. For example, if a patient has lung cancer, a chest CT scan alone will not give a clear picture of the patient's liver. If a patient has colorectal cancer without known lung metastases, then a CT scan of the abdomen and pelvis plus a chest x-ray should provide the needed baseline information. If the chest x-ray indicates possible metastasis, however, then a CT of the chest should also be ordered. Unless a patient has known bone metastasis or is complaining of bone pain, a bone scan is not generally ordered. Likewise, if a patient has no history of brain metastasis and no symptoms suggesting brain metastasis, a brain scan is not ordered. On the other hand, a patient with renal cell carcinoma, because of the natural course of the disease, should have CTs of the chest, abdomen, and pelvis as well as a bone scan. Always discuss appropriate screening exams with the principal investigator.

Tumor Markers

Tumor markers are blood tests that *may* be indicators of certain diseases. Some tumor markers are specific to a certain cancer; for example, OV125 is specific to ovarian cancer and PSA is specific to prostate cancer. Other tumor markers may be elevated in a variety of cancers; for example, carcinoembryonic antigen (CEA) can be related to breast cancer, lung cancer, and several gastrointestinal cancers. However, not every cancer has a specific tumor marker and not every patient with a specific type of cancer will necessarily have an elevation of the tumor marker. When appropriate, a tumor marker is a relatively inexpensive, noninvasive means of following disease. Be aware that a tumor marker may be very high with very little disease seen on a CT scan and, conversely, a CT scan may reveal lots of tumor burden with a very low or even normal tumor marker.

Nonetheless, if the diagnosis is associated with a tumor marker, a tumor marker should be drawn and recorded at baseline. At the beginning of every cycle of treatment, the tumor marker must be repeated. Be aware that no treatment decisions are based on tumor markers alone. Still, a rising tumor marker may suggest that disease is progressing and can guide restaging decisions.

Baseline Laboratory Tests

The time requirement for screening lab work is usually within 7 to 10 days of starting the study drug. Consult the protocol to be sure. Screening labs always include a complete blood count, with differential and platelet count, and a chemistry panel. The definition of a chemistry panel varies from sponsor to sponsor and study to study, so check the protocol. The protocol typically includes an appendix that defines the required laboratory tests. Don't forget to draw the appropriate tumor marker and, if necessary, a pregnancy test. Some protocols call for serum pregnancy tests while others will allow a urine pregnancy test; know what your protocol requires.

Baseline labs might require other blood tests, such as flow cytometry, that are specific to a certain study. Generally, a baseline urinalysis is also required.

A baseline prothrombin time (PT) and activate partial thromboplastin time (APTT) might also be needed. Carefully read the appendix that outlines the needed blood tests to be sure that everything the sponsor requires has been included on your requisition.

Calculating Lab Values

Sometimes calculations are required to determine certain lab values. For example, the absolute neutrophil count (ANC) is essential to determine whether it is safe to give a patient more treatment with a drug that causes myelosuppression. An ANC that is too low might put the patient at risk if he or she contracts an infection and lacks sufficient neutrophils to mount a response. Some labs only report neutrophils as a percentage. In such a case, multiply the total white blood count (WBC) by the percent of neutrophils to determine the absolute neutrophil count. For example, if WBC is 5.2 and the percent of neutrophils is 55.1, then

$$\text{WBC} \times \text{Neutrophils} = \text{ANC}$$

$$5.2 \times 0.551 = 2.9$$

Other lab values that may require calculations include the globulin (G), which is the total protein minus the albumin (A). The A/G ratio is determined by dividing the albumin by the globulin. Some studies ask for the total bilirubin and the indirect bilirubin. Laboratories can measure the total bilirubin and the direct bilirubin (or conjugated bilirubin). The *indirect bilirubin* is then determined by subtracting the direct bilirubin from the total bilirubin. If such calculations are required, a letter to file (that is, a memo placed in the regulatory binder) may be needed to document how you arrived at the numbers in question.

$$\text{T. Protein} - \text{Albumin} = \text{Globulin}$$

$$\text{Albumin/Globulin} = \text{A/G Ratio}$$

$$\text{T. Bilirubin} - \text{D. Bilirubin} = \text{Indirect Bilirubin}$$

Scrutinizing Lab Values

Be sure to carefully scrutinize all of the results. If there are abnormal values reported in labs other than those required for entry to the study, they may affect the patient's ability to participate in the study. For example, if a patient is hypercalcemic (elevated serum calcium) or hypokalemic (low potassium level), these problems may need to be addressed *before* the patient starts the study drug. If an abnormal value may be an error (for example, a prolonged PTT that was drawn from a heparinized line), run the test again to clarify whether there really is an abnormality in the patient's labs or a technical error in obtaining or processing the specimen *before* the patient starts the study drug.

> **Note**
>
> Some protocols require that once a patient is consented, registered, and randomized (if applicable) as a participant—even if he or she *never* receives the drug—the patient must be followed for **intent to treat**. Usually this requires baseline data and follow-up survival information.

Baseline Signs and Symptoms

An in-depth review of the patient's current symptoms at baseline is essential to identifying and grading adverse events later in the trial. These *subjective* baseline symptoms will *not* be noted on the *objective* physical exam—for example, fatigue, pain, and paresthesia. Some CRFs include a page for this information. The physical exam at baseline also must encompass all physical findings. Be sure to assign a grade to these signs and symptoms. If a page is not provided for baseline signs and symptoms, then record the information in the Past Medical History section.

Recording the objective findings of a physical examination can sometimes be difficult for data entry staff who are not clinically oriented. Provide guidelines to help ensure accurate recording (Appendix A). Handwriting might be difficult to decipher and so, too, might be certain symbols and abbreviations that are not universally understood. An example of one such abbreviation is ∅c/c/e, which means no cyanosis, clubbing, or edema.

Any new physical findings that develops during the study should be noted as an adverse event. Any finding on the baseline physical exam should be noted at each subsequent physical exam; omission of it at a later exam will be interpreted as resolution of the original finding. Therefore, it is useful to have the most recent physical exam report available during the current visit to ensure that all previous findings, if not resolved, are again noted.

Helpful Hint

Record all of the screening data as soon *after* the patient has started the study as possible. *After* is the operative word here. Anything can happen to interfere with the patient starting the study, so do not take the chance of wasting time to study and record the patient's history until you are sure that he or she is going to participate in the trial.

■ Treatment Data

If your orders allow for prn (as needed) medications to be administered, be sure that the treating nurse indicates on the order what is given, why it is given, and what the outcome is. For example, if the patient experienced nausea during the treatment and was given prochlorperazine maleate (Compazine) with resolution of the symptom, the nausea must be recorded as an adverse event and the prochlorperazine maleate must be recorded as a concomitant medication.

The most important and challenging part of recording the treatment data can be getting the orders completed and returned from the treatment area. Keep close track of the orders. If orders are missing, they are usually much easier to find sooner rather than later. Just like outside records, if an order goes down to the medical records department as a loose sheet of paper, it may be like looking for a needle in a haystack. When you receive the completed orders, review each item to ensure that it is filled out completely and logically. Be vigilant. For example, a drug administration start time of 1400 and stop time of 1130 should alert you to a problem.

Adverse Events

Any sign or symptom that the patient experiences during the course of the study is classified an adverse event even if you are certain it is not related to the study drug. Differentiating between a baseline symptom and something new can be challenging. When a patient is telling you about fatigue or pain, you must ask, "Is this different from what you felt before starting the study drug?" If a sign or symptom that was present at baseline becomes worse, it must be recorded as an adverse event but at a higher grade than was present at baseline.

All abnormal lab results must be recorded as adverse events unless they are believed not to be clinically significant. For example, if you see a blood urea nitrogen (BUN) of 21 and the high side of normal is

20, you would probably not consider that finding clinically significant. An exception would be if the sponsor observed renal failure in the animal studies. In that case, the sponsor will have low tolerance for abnormalities in renal function and would most likely ask that all such irregularities be recorded. If in doubt, consult the monitor or the principal investigator.

The study coordinator or the data manager should see the patient at each visit, review ongoing adverse events, and record any adverse events that the patient may have experienced since the last visit. Encouraging the patient to keep a diary helps track such information. A recent study on adverse event reporting looked at a variety of methods used to collect this information. It concluded that patient diaries yielded significantly more adverse events than other forms of assessment.[3]

The event should be graded according to the National Cancer Institute (NCI) toxicity scale. The NCI toxicity tables, called the Common Toxicity Criteria (CTC), were updated in 1998 and are now quite detailed. However, if the table fails to cover a specific adverse event, the event should be graded as mild (1), moderate (2), severe (3), life-threatening (4), or fatal (5). Be extremely careful when assigning these subjective gradings. You must try to interpret *subjective* symptoms in an *objective* manner. If a patient describes severe fatigue, determine whether the patient has been unable to get out of bed since the last treatment or if a 1-hour nap relieved the symptom.

Adverse events that are graded III or higher are generally defined as serious adverse events. Particularly in phase I studies, a grade 3 adverse event may be viewed as a dose-limiting toxicity and require alterations in accrual or to completely stop the study. If you are considering classifying an event as a grade 3, consult the principal investigator. If it is clear that a grade 3 toxicity has occurred, inform the principal investigator immediately. Often, grade 3 or 4 laboratory toxicities will *not* be dose-limiting, particularly in patients who did not have a normal value at baseline. Do not guess; when in doubt, review the numbers with the investigator.

Serious Adverse Events

A serious adverse event (SAE) is one that results in any of the following outcomes: death, a life-threatening adverse event, inpatient hospitalization or prolongation of existing hospitalization, a persistent or significant disability/incapacity, or a congenital abnormality. Serious adverse events must be reported to the sponsor with 24 hours of your knowledge of the event. Inform the sponsor's drug safety officer by phone, then complete the SAE form provided by the sponsor. These forms vary but, typically, they ask for the facts surrounding the event, some pertinent background information, concomitant medications, and causality regarding the study medication. Tell the whole story but be succinct. Attach supporting labs, radiology reports, admission history and physical, consults—whatever information you have available. The study coordinator must complete this form and secure the principal investigator's signature. Alternatively, a coinvestigator may sign the SAE, but be sure to inform the principal investigator about the incident.

Fax the completed, signed SAE form to the sponsor and make three copies; distribute as follows:

- Place the original in the patient's CRF.
- File one copy with the institutional review board (IRB).
- Place one copy in the patient's research chart.
- Retain one copy for filing the final report.

Note: When the SAE has been filed with the IRB, a copy of the SAE and the IRB reporting form must be placed in the regulatory binder.

Report SAEs Promptly

Reporting SAEs are your highest priority after patient care. Typically, an SAE must be reported to the IRB within a specific time frame, such as 5 working days. If the SAE is death on study (even if not related to the study drug), it generally must be reported to the IRB within 24 hours.

Obtain Hospital Records

If the patient is hospitalized, obtain hospital records and record all medications and associated adverse events that occur during hospitalization. For example, the patient may experience hypokalemia while hospitalized and receive a potassium supplement. Record the hypokalemia as an AE and the potassium as a concomitant medication. If the patient is hospitalized at your facility, copy the chart every few days or make copies right after the patient is discharged and before the chart goes to the medical records department. If you do not promptly secure the information, the chart may be kept in discharge analysis or utilization review for several weeks while all dictations, signatures, and insurance issues are resolved.

Closing Out and Tracking the SAE

When the patient is discharged or the SAE is otherwise resolved, close out the SAE. Update a copy of the original SAE by adding outcome information, the discharge summary, and any other pertinent results, and send it to the sponsor and the IRB.

Always track SAEs. This process is critical for two reasons. First, particularly in a phase I trial, careful records will help you discern whether a trend or pattern, possibly related to the study drug, is developing. Second, tracking allows you to monitor the filing status of each SAE. Has a follow-up or final report been filed for each event? During monitoring or auditing, this log is quite helpful (Figure 11–2).

MedWatch Reporting

Whenever an SAE occurs that is determined to be related or that may be related to the study drug, the sponsor must file a MedWatch report with the U.S. Food and Drug Administration (FDA). The form is designed to give the FDA pertinent details of the event. The sponsor completes the form which is provided by the FDA and sends a copy of the report to all sites that have used or are using that drug. In phase II or phase III trials, hundreds of sites might be involved. All MedWatch reports must also be filed with the IRB; usually a simple cover letter is sufficient. However, the principal investigator may decide to draft a letter with a more detailed explanation if the situation warrants it.

If the event described had not previously been identified as a possible side effect, the sponsor will likely prepare a protocol amendment. The amendment must be filed with the IRB and changes to the informed consent made. While awaiting a new, IRB-approved consent that all patients must sign, inform study participants of the new finding, and document this discussion in your progress notes.

Confusion may result if the SAE that triggered the MedWatch report occurred at your site. Though the original event report has been filed with your IRB, the MedWatch report must be filed as well. Track the filing of the MedWatch reports (Figure 11–3), and preserve this record for use during an audit.

■ End of Study

If restaging indicates that a patient has progressed, he or she will be terminated from the study. Be sure to check the protocol for tests that must be done at end of study. The end-of-study date is usually the date the physician reviews the results of the restaging with the patient and officially removes the patient from the study. A note must be written indicating the plan to be "off study." The investigator must document why the patient is being taken off study to avoid confusion during the monitoring process.

SAE Tracking Log

STUDY NAME _____

IRB # _____

#	SERIOUS ADVERSE EVENT	PT INITIALS	PT NUMBER	PRELIM REPORT rec'd	to IRB	FOLLOW-UP REPORT rec'd	to IRB	FINAL REPORT rec'd	to IRB	COMMENTS

Figure 11–2 Sample SAE tracking log

MedWatch Tracking Log

STUDY NAME _____

IRB # _____

MEDWATCH	DATE RECEIVED	DATE SENT TO IRB

Figure 11–3 Sample MedWatch tracking log

101

Radiographic evidence of disease progression is only one criterion for termination from study. Patients may demonstrate clinical signs of progression, such as extreme fatigue, cachexia, or other manifestations, that cause a significant decline in their performance status. Occasionally, patients choose to withdraw their consent and, in effect, remove themselves from the study. They may be concerned about a side effect seen in another patient or they may simply be tired of receiving treatment.

At times, patients are taken off study retrospectively. For example, if treatment was temporarily interrupted due to an adverse event that was later determined to be progressive disease, the patient's off-study date could revert to the date when the clinical symptoms of progression were first noted. The off-study date should *not* be the last date that the patient received the drug. It may, however, be the next day.

The off-study date is important because all adverse events, serious adverse events, and deaths occurring within 30 days of that date must be reported as if the patient were still receiving the study medication. If a patient dies more than 30 days after coming off study, only a death report must be filed with the sponsor.

Follow-up

A follow-up evaluation is generally required 30 days after the patient has come off study. A physical exam, performance status, and labs are usually required. At this point, all ongoing adverse events should be resolved or indicated to be continuing. All concomitant medications also must be reviewed and given either stop dates or classified as continuing. If an adverse event that has been coded related to the study drug is still ongoing at the 30-day follow-up visit, the sponsor will require that the adverse event be followed until resolution. If the AE has continued for 30 days after the drug was stopped, reconsider the relationship to the study drug. The AE is probably related to the underlying disease.

Mark the calendar for 30 days after the patient comes off study, and prepare ahead. Follow-up visits can be done from 2 to 6 weeks after the last dose of the study drug. Check the protocol. Generally, the sponsor is fairly lenient about this time point because some data are better, even if out of their specified window, than no data at all.

If the patient cannot return to your facility because of distance or poor performance status, obtain the necessary information from the patient's current (off-study) treating physician. Be clear about what you need. Fax copies of the CRF pages, if necessary, to assist the outside physician to provide the complete information.

■ Comments

Most CRFs include a comment section for recording any irregularity in the treatment, such as a missing vital sign or lab result or anything that may need clarification. Detailed explanations are not needed in most cases; be concise and succinct. Noting that a vital sign was inadvertently missed is sufficient. You do not need to explain that there was an emergency with another patient or that a lab technician dropped a tube. If the patient has abnormal lab values at baseline, note them here, "grade 1 anemia and grade 1 alkaline phosphatase at baseline." If day 21 labs were actually drawn on day 22 because of a holiday, write a comment. If the design of the CRF does not allow you to tell the whole story, add a comment for clarification. It is better to add a comment and avoid a query than to not have commented at all!

Remember that the CRF should tell the story of what happened to the patient while part of the study. Use the comment section to fill any gaps in information. Using your comment section wisely can save hours of corrections and queries in the end.

■ Missing or Unknown Data

Despite the many discussions about completing the CRFs you will have had with the monitor, some small but troubling questions always seem to crop up, such as:

- If information has been requested that cannot be found (for example, exact dates of prior therapies), shall I write "unknown," or use dashes, or use zeros?
- Shall I use Not Done (ND) or Not Available (NA) if there is a lab value that the lab does not run (for example, urobilinogen in a urinalysis)?

If the monitor's first visit is scheduled for shortly after the enrollment of the first patient, these questions can probably wait until then. If there is a delay in the first monitoring visit, however, waiting to ask questions could result in a lot of avoidable corrections. Instead, ask these questions up front at the site initiation visit.

■ Tracking Data

A data tracking form (Figure 11–4) has many uses. If more than one person is working on the study, the form can be kept at the front

Data Tracking Form

PATIENT _____   STUDY _____

Cycle, Week	Completed	Monitored	CRF Pulled	PKs Sent	Comments

Figure 11-4 Sample data tracking form

of the CRF as a helpful reference. The form also helps when preparing for a monitoring visit. In a single glance, you can spot what may be incomplete or missing. Use the comment section of this form to track requests for outside records.

■ References

1. *Southwest Oncology Group Clinical Research Manual.* (1999). Vol. I, Chapter 7. 7-2–7-11.
2. Therasse, P., Arbuck, S. G., Eisenhauer, E. A., Wanders, J., Kaplan, R. S., Rubenstein, L., et al. (2000). New guidelines to evaluate the response to treatment in solid tumors. *Journal of the National Cancer Institute* 92(3), 205–216.
3. Edwards, J. E., McQuay, H. J., Moore, R. A., & Collins, S. L. (1999). Reporting of adverse events in clinical trials should be improved: Lessons from acute postoperative pain. *Journal of Pain and Symptom Management,* 18(6), 427–437.

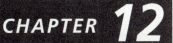

CHAPTER 12

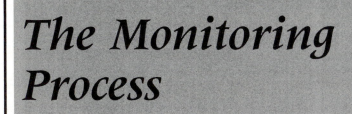

The Monitoring Process

■ The Monitor

The sponsor has the responsibility to verify that all regulatory procedures are followed, drug is accounted for, and the data is correct. The sponsor's designee is known as the study monitor and may be either an employee of the sponsor or someone contracted by the sponsor. Occasionally, pharmaceutical companies arrange for a contract research organization (CRO) to manage a clinical trial. In such cases, all regulatory documents are sent to the CRO, and the monitor is employed by the CRO; this arrangement adds an extra layer of authority between the study site and the sponsor. Alternatively, the sponsor may hire an independent contractor to monitor the trial. The monitor will report directly to the project manager at the sponsor. Whatever the organizational structure, the monitoring process is the same.

■ Visit Frequency and Overview

Soon after the first patient is enrolled, expect the monitor to schedule a monitoring visit. If the monitor does not schedule a visit just after the first patient has been accrued, call the monitor and request a visit. Though you will be working busily on case report forms (CRFs),

105

it is best to get early input about how the data are to recorded, which will clarify the monitor's expectations and save time.

After the initial visit, and depending on the accrual, the monitor will return every 1 to 2 months. Some visits may require 1 day and others 1 week or more, depending on the number of patients accrued during that time period and the amount of outstanding data.

Letter of Intent

Once the date of the monitoring visit has been set, the monitor sends a letter stating which patients' data will be monitored. This letter should arrive in plenty of time for the patients' medical records to be retrieved and for all current data to be brought up-to-date.

Letter of Follow-up

Following the monitoring visit, the monitor again sends a letter, this time stating what was monitored, what corrections are still outstanding, and when the next monitoring visit will occur. Any required corrections should be addressed as soon after the visit as possible. Just prior to the monitor's next visit, review this letter to ensure that all requested corrections have been made. File letters from the monitor under Study Communication in the regulatory binder; they are excellent records and provide valuable reference in case of an audit.

The Common Goal

Monitoring visits should *not* be adversarial. Both you and the monitor have the same goal—accurate data.

Bear in mind that, when it comes to data collection and recording, every sponsor is different; and that every study, even when run by the same sponsor, is different; and that each monitor from that sponsor is unique. It is important to come to a meeting of the minds about completing the CRFs. If the monitor asks you to do something that does not make sense to you, you may want to clarify it with the sponsor's project manager or discuss it with the principal investigator.

The lack of standardization in approach that plagues study coordinators also affects study monitors. Be patient, and listen to what the monitor is saying. Each new monitor can be a source of new information.

■ Preparing for the Visit

To prepare for a monitoring visit, carefully review every page of each CRF requested to ensure that all data are complete. Always do this *before* presenting a CRF to the monitor. The monitor must see the patient's outpatient medical record, inpatient medical record (if applicable), the research chart, and the CRF. Be sure to allow yourself enough time to retrieve the charts from the medical records department *before* the monitor's visit. Recall that the research chart is *not* the source document.

The monitor will also need the regulatory binder(s) at each visit. If you file materials promptly and regularly, this should not present a problem. Be sure all tracking logs and screening logs are up-to-date prior to the monitor's visit as well. The monitor will sign the monitoring log each time he or she visits the site.

■ Data Corrections

The monitor checks the data in the medical records and research chart against the CRF to verify that all data have been correctly recorded. No matter how careful you are, there *will* be corrections. There are *always* corrections so do not take corrections as a failure on your part.

Occasionally, the monitor may ask you to make a change that doesn't seem to make sense or appropriate to you. See if you can resolve the issue with discussion. Depending on the seriousness of your concern, you may want to seek input from the principal investigator. If the matter is not significant, record the information as requested. The monitor may have knowledge of an incident at another site that prompts the request. For example, the sponsor may have noted a decrease in several patients' phosphorus levels. Although such a change would not usually be considered significant, the sponsor will want all changes tracked to try to determine if the study drug is implicated.

There is a proper way to make corrections. Place a single line through an error, then record the correct information, date it, and initial it (Figure 12–1). *Never* white out, erase, or black out an error. Also, be sure to write legibly using black ink. Do not write so large that there is no room for additional corrections, if needed. Do not write so small that the correction is illegible; illegible entries will generate queries.

If the CRF has multiple copies, be sure that the entries are legible on all copies. If not, trying to read the data when answering queries will be impossible.

■ Pulling the Data

When the data has been monitored and corrected, two things happen: (1) you get paid, and (2) data are compiled in an electronic database.

Incorrect	**Correct**
~~12~~	~~12~~——mdm 3/1/00
	21
☞	
~~90 mdm~~	~~90~~ mdm 3/1/00
	09
~~Tiral~~	~~Tiral~~ mdm 3/1/00
	Trial

Figure 12–1 The proper way to make a data correction.

Payment may be contingent on the sponsor receiving data, so it is important to get the data completed, monitored, and corrected in a timely fashion. Use a tracking form so that you or your financial department are aware what the next invoice should cover. (See Table 4–2 for a sample tracking form.)

The corrected data are sent by the monitor for entry into an electronic database. Usually the CRF pages are NCR paper allowing the monitor to *pull* (remove) the top one or two pages, leaving at least one copy in the book. Some CRFs may be single, barcoded pages that are faxed directly to the company that has been contracted to manage the database. The computer matches and cross-checks all of the entries to determine whether something is missing or does not match; it then generates queries if discrepancies are found.

■ Queries

Any queries about the data are sent to the test site for clarification. Early queries are usually simple: missed check marks, vital signs out of range, or adverse events that do not match with concomitant medications. As the database grows, the queries may become more complex until the data are finalized. If your first response to a query did not clarify the issue, expect follow-up queries.

The sponsor gives data rules to the data management company. These data rules define parameters for clinical significance of vital signs and lab values. Occasionally, issues that arise in the queries may need further clarification by the sponsor. Don't hesitate to contact the monitor or project manager if you are being asked to make corrections that do not make sense to you or to correct things that you believe were recorded correctly in the first place. And always be certain that you understand what a query is asking. Clarifying these issues with the sponsor early on will save time and improve your understanding of the sponsor's expectations. Queries are actually a good exercise in learning to record clean data.

■ Audits

If there is one word that strikes fear in the heart of a study coordinator, it is the word AUDIT!!! At various times, either during a study or after a study is closed, an **audit** might be announced. An audit may be conducted randomly or it may be called for cause, meaning that something has brought your site or study to the attention of the auditing body. There are several types of audits that a study may be subjected to:

- A *quality-assurance audit* is an internal process in which the quality assurance committee of the institutional review board (IRB) reviews study procedures and data collection to ensure that all patient treatment and data are in compliance with the protocol, IRB regulations, and the FDA. Such an audit usually occurs while the study is in progress.
- A *sponsor-driven audit* is initiated by the sponsor to confirm that the trial has been run according to the protocol, data have been recorded and monitored correctly, and that the regulatory binder is complete. A sponsor-driven audit is usually prompted by anticipation of an FDA audit. If the data have been recorded and monitored in a timely manner and the regulatory binder has been kept current, this audit will require little work on your part.
- An *FDA audit* is a federal action initiated by the FDA. This type of audit is common in phase III trials as an investigational drug is nearing approval. The sites to be audited are generally determined by accrual; if your site has the highest accrual on a specific study, expect an FDA audit.

    The FDA investigates all aspects of protocol compliance, patient accrual and consent, data collection, and drug accountability. Though an FDA audit can be somewhat nerve-racking, attention to detail throughout in the protocol's execution will make this audit less difficult. Preparing for an FDA audit is no different than preparing for a quality-assurance audit.

In all audits, the auditor will request access to the regulatory binder and CRFs and original source documents for specific patients. The number of charts requested will range from 10 to 50 percent of the total number of patients accrued. The auditor may thoroughly review some charts and spot-check others. If the auditor discovers a problem in one chart, he or she may review every chart to determine whether the problem was consistent. Although the auditor originally requests specific patient records, he or she is free to request, at any time, the records of *every* patient treated on the trial.

Preparing for an Audit

To prepare for any audit, carefully review the regulatory binder for the following items:

- Copies of the original protocol and all amendments
- Copies of all consents used during the trial (all must show the IRB approval stamp)
- All IRB approval letters
- Copies of letters reporting all serious adverse events (SAEs) to the IRB
- Copies of the letters reporting all MedWatches to the IRB
- All correspondence with the sponsor (including any letters of exception given during the trial)
- The signature page that includes signatures of all investigators and any other personnel who worked on the trial
- The monitoring log that the monitors signed at each visit
- Pharmacy dispensing and drug accountability logs

The SAE and MedWatch logs are critical during an audit. If you have any doubt about whether the regulatory binder contains all such reports, consult the sponsor to confirm that your files agree.

Carefully review all of the medical records to be certain that the documentation is complete. It is extremely useful (and will give you points with the auditor) to flag the important documents in each medical record for the auditor's easy reference. The auditor will examine the original consent to ensure that the patient was consented prior to initiating any screening procedures; likewise, all documentation of the screening will be reviewed to confirm that the patient was indeed eligible for the trial. By flagging screening labs, baseline radiographic studies (if the study calls for measurable disease), the pathology report, and the screening visit, you will help expedite the auditor's review. If your study required repeat radiographic studies at specific intervals for continuation on the study, flag each restaging CT or x-ray so that the auditor can easily follow the progress of each patient.

Protocol Violations

The auditor looks for protocol violations. Even in the best-run study, a protocol violation may occur. If, during the study, you become aware that your site has committed a protocol violation, notify the sponsor immediately and be sure to document that notification. Ideally, any protocol misstep were found by the monitor and corrected or addressed during the study. However, this is not always the case.

If, while reviewing data prior to the audit, you find a problem, do *not* change the CRF. The problem must be addressed in current time. For example, if you find that a CT scan suggests a new lesion that might be progressive disease, but the investigator chose to continue the patient on trial, there must be a progress note in the record clearly explaining the investigator's rationale. If the proper note was not written when this occurred and not corrected when the data was initially reviewed, the investigator must write the note after the fact, date it, and place it in the patient's medical record.

Important Note

An audit is the proverbial moment of truth. The process can be a very useful learning tool that will help you to identify any deficiencies in your procedures. Careful, clear, and accurate documentation and data collection from the start will make preparing for an audit far less difficult in the end.

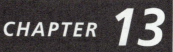
Closing the Study

When all of the data have been collected, the CRFs monitored, the corrections made, and the queries answered (yes, it will really happen), just a few housekeeping issues remain. You should advise the investigational pharmacy and the IRB that the study is officially closed.

■ Drug Disposal

At the end of a study, the sponsor must dispose of any remaining drug. The sponsor might retrieve the drug or arrange with the pharmacist to destroy it. Though these arrangements are made between the sponsor and the pharmacy, it must be documented as part of the study communication. If there are any remaining CRFs and lab kits, ask the sponsor what should be done with them.

■ Document Storage

Keep the CRFs and research charts close at hand until the study's final report has been filed with the FDA. Once the final report has been submitted, collect all CRFs, regulatory binders, and research charts and send them to a storage facility.

FDA regulations mandate that records be retained for a specific time period. For investigational new drug studies, records are kept for 2 years after marketing application approval has been granted to the drug for the indication studied in that particular trial. If no application is filed, or if the application is not approved, the records will be retained for 2 years after the study is closed.

Reminder

Investigators should request that study sponsors keep them informed about the status of the applications for studies that they conducted.

When you have completed all of this, take yourself out to lunch and bask in the glory for a few minutes. The next study is waiting for you.

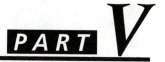
PART V

Organizational Issues

- *Organizing a Research Program*

- *Standard Operating Procedures*

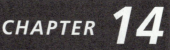

Organizing a Research Program

Research programs can vary in size from a small program of one investigator and one study coordinator to a large, complicated program having multiple physicians, study coordinators, data managers, and support staff. No matter what the program's size or complexity, the steps for coordinating and conducting a clinical trial that are outlined in the preceding chapters can be applied.

■ Small Program—Heavy Workload

If the program is small, the study coordinator may be responsible for *everything*, including filing regulatory documents, writing budgets, recruiting patients, collecting and recording data, as well as handling monitoring visits, and answering queries. Such an arrangement will obviously limit the number of clinical trials that can be done. Workload issues related to the phase of the study must also be considered. For example, if a phase I study is being run, the study coordinator will collect and ship pharmacokinetic (PK) samples in addition to the exhaustive list of duties previously noted.

■ Larger Program—More Balanced Workload

In a large program, common organizational structure includes a data manager, an investigator, and a study coordinator. The way responsibilities are divided between the study coordinator and the data manager is determined by a number of variables. Past experience in clinical trials, acuity of patients, and the rate of accrual are just a few of the things to consider when dividing duties. Most frequently, the data manager is responsible for preparing the institutional review board (IRB) filing and recording data. Depending on the clinical expertise of the data manager, he or she may need the study coordinator's assistance in interpreting and recording adverse events and laboratory and CT results. This division of responsibility will allow the team to handle more clinical trials.

■ Hiring Personnel

Often, as programs grow, the need for additional personnel arises. Should more study coordinators or more data managers be hired? The characteristics of the program will most likely dictate the need. For example, if several phase I studies are being conducted, another nurse study coordinator may be needed to provide good clinical coverage for the more acute patient population. Typically, having more data managers and support staff allows the nurse to see more patients—a definite benefit.

■ Decentralizing Responsibilities

If the program is large, consider decentralizing responsibilities. Hiring one person to handle all regulatory affairs may be more efficient than requiring each study coordinator or data manager to oversee these aspects of their studies. A dedicated regulatory person will be an expert in regulatory affairs and can focus on filing and tracking documents with the IRB.

Likewise, it may be prudent to make one person responsible for writing and negotiating budgets, and tracking payments and expenditures. The more trials you conduct, the more complicated it becomes to stay on top of finances. Careful financial management is essential to the success of your program.

Some investigators want to manage the research program; others prefer to delegate day-to-day management decisions. The investigator's experience in clinical research and any other commitments will dictate his or her ability to be involved in the details.

Strive for Clarity

Whatever the structure, be sure that everyone involved in the research program understands the division of labor and who is responsible for what. In a very busy program, responsibilities may need to be changed as the workload shifts. Do not find out the day before the monitor comes out that no one has filed that last amendment to the protocol or that the data manager thought you were maintaining the regulatory binder. Excellent personnel, good management, and clear direction and flexibility are key to a well-run research program.

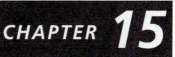

Standard Operating Procedures

Standard operating procedures (SOP) are a good idea no matter what the size of your program. The larger the program, however, the more important it is to have written SOPs in place.

Mission Statement

Every program should have a mission statement. Sitting down with your investigator and discussing your common vision and goals helps to clarify a program's priorities and direction. Defining your goals will assure that everyone in your program is starting on the same page and working with a clear sense of purpose.

Site Administration

Another SOP should define the site administration. A simple organization chart can delineate lines of authority and responsibility. It might look something like Figure 15–1.

121

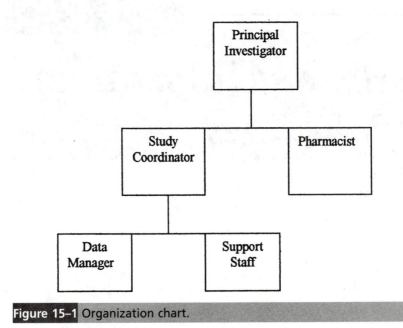

Figure 15–1 Organization chart.

■ Other Documentation

In most organizations, SOPs are already in place for drug management issues. Likewise, written policies and procedures are probably in place to define procedures used in the treatment area.

A written statement about your program's compliance with Good Clinical Practice, like all other documentation, helps everyone involved understand the principles and comply with them. After the roles and responsibilities of the staff members have been established, describe staff functions and job requirements in SOPs.

The larger the team, the more important it is to have well-written SOPs. If the research program grows quickly, it may be difficult to keep up with the changes, and the need for SOPs becomes even more critical.

Perseverance is a great element of success.
If you only knock long enough and
loud enough at the gate,
you are sure to wake up somebody.

Henry Wadsworth Longfellow

Appendixes

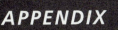

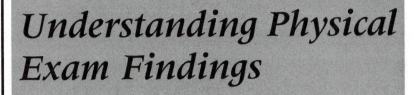

Understanding Physical Exam Findings

Physical exam findings are always *objective*. The symptoms the patient describes (for example, fatigue or shortness of breath) are listed under review of systems (ROS) on the progress note and are *subjective*.

Here are some common entries you may find recorded under physical exam:

HEENT = Head, eyes, ears, nose, and throat
Normal
Anicteric
PERRL (pupils, equal round and reactive to light)
Oropharynx or nasopharynx clear

Abnormal
Mucositis (mouth sores or ulcers)
Alopecia (loss of hair)

Nodes = Lymph nodes
Abnormal
If positive will describe location (e.g., supraclavicular, axillary) and sometimes size in cm

Chest
Normal
CTA = Clear to auscultation (listening)
Abnormal
Rales, rhonchi, or wheezing heard in either lung or both lungs (bilateral) or bases

CV = Cardiovascular (this relates not only to the heart but also to the blood vessels; a central venous access device would be listed under CV, not chest)
Normal
RRR = Regular rate and rhythm
NSR = Normal sinus rhythm
S_1, S_2
Abnormal
Tachycardia = HR > 100
Bradycardia = HR < 60
Split S_1
SM = Systolic murmur (a leaking heart valve)

Abdomen
Normal
Soft, ∅ tender, + BS (bowel sounds)
Neither the liver or spleen are palpable
Abnormal
Hypoactive or hyperactive bowel sounds
+ HM (Hepatomegaly; enlarged liver); usually noted to be XXcm below RCM (right costal margin) or XX FB (fingerbreaths) below RCM.
+ Splenomegaly (enlarged spleen); would be below LCM (left costal margin)

Extremities
Normal
∅ c/c/e = No clubbing, cyanosis, or edema
Abnormal
Clubbing noted in fingertips
Cyanosis noted in nailbeds
Edema can be described as 1+, 2+, etc., and location
    BLE = bilateral lower extremities
    LLE = left lower extremity
    RLE = right lower extremity

Peripheral neuropathy = numbness, tingling usually in fingers, and/or toes; sometimes called paresthesia

Neurological
Normal
Nonfocal
Abnormal
Can include weakness of an extremity, difficulty with vision, speech, thought processes

Skin
Normal
Clear
Abnormal
Rashes (macular, papular, redness, petechiae (tiny, flat red bumps)
Lesions (closed or open)
Ecchymosis (bruising)

Musculoskeletal
Abnormal
Myalgias (muscle aches)
Arthralgias (joint aches)
Tenderness

Electronic Resources

The World Wide Web can provide a wealth of information to health care professionals and patients. With a computer, modem, and Internet account, information on a multitude of subjects can be accessed in a few minutes. The Internet resources listed here may provide helpful information to you and your patients.

The National Cancer Institute has many Web sites to disseminate information to both health care professionals and the public. Below are several resources that you may find helpful.

Physician Data Query (PDQ®)—a comprehensive database containing information on all aspects of cancer care including summaries of over 1,500 current clinical trials. *http://cancernet.nci.nih.gov/pdq.htm* cancerTrials™ is a new resource which is a comprehensive listing of clinical trials. *http://cancertrials.nci.nih.gov/*
Common toxicity criteria is available online. *http://ctep.info.nih.gov*

The U.S. Food and Drug Administration (FDA) also has several Web sites that may be useful to your organization.

The FDA Home Page is located at *www.fda.gov/*
The FDA Cancer Liaison Program Home Page at *www.fda.gov/oashi/ cancer/cancer.html*

The Good Clinical Practice Guidelines (GCP) can be found at *www.fda
.gov/cder*

You can also visit the Web sites of several professional organizations:

Association of Clinical Research Professionals (ACRP) is an international association of research professionals with a goal of professional
growth. *www.acrpnet.org*

Drug Information Association (DIA) is an international, scientific association. *www.diahome.org*

Oncology Nursing Society is a national organization of registered
nurses and other health care professionals involved in the field of
oncology. Within that organization are several special interest
groups including the Clinical Trial Nurses. *www.ons.org*

Society of Clinical Research Associates, Inc. (SoCRA) is an organization
of clinical research associates and other health care professionals.
www.socra.com

Glossary

Absolute neutrophil count The exact number of neutrophils; determined by multiplying the total white blood count by the percentage of neutrophils; generally required to be >1.5 to give a patient cytotoxic drugs

Adjuvant therapy Treatment given after surgical resection when no objective evidence of remaining disease exists

Adverse event Any change experienced by a study subject after enrolling in a clinical trial

AE See adverse event

Amendment A change or addition to the original protocol

ANC See Absolute neutrophil count

Arm In a comparative study, different therapies are defined as arms

Audit A careful review of study data, protocol procedures, study conduct, and/or outcomes to verify that the data is correct and that procedures have been carried out properly

Baseline Measurements (laboratory results, tumor measurements) taken prior to starting study procedures and used to determine response to study treatment

Bidimensional measurements Measurements of the two dimensions of lesions seen on a Radiographic Study

Bioavailability Determination of the amount of drug, or its metabolites, that is detectable in the patient's serum

Blinded study A randomized study in which neither the research team nor the patient knows which treatment the patient is receiving; the purpose is to avoid bias

Body surface area A calculation using the patient's height and weight; used to determine treatment dose in some studies

Breach of contract When one party does not meet the terms of the contract

BSA See body surface area

CAP College of Pathologists (laboratory certification)

Carcinogen A substance that causes cancer

Case report form Documents used to record data gathered during the course of a clinical trial

Causality Relationship between an adverse event and the study drug

Chemotherapy A chemical compound used to treat a symptom or disease

CLIA Clinical Laboratory Improvement Amendments (laboratory certification)

Clinical research coordinator A health care professional who is responsible for the organization and execution of study activities

Clinical trial A research study to test drugs or devices in humans

Cohort A group of patients who all receive the same dose of a drug in a phase I clinical trial

Coinvestigator A physician or other qualified individual who assists the principal investigator in executing the protocol

Common Toxicity Criteria Table used to quantify toxicities

Contract A legal document that is executed between the principal investigator and the sponsor, defining their agreement on publication rights, financial matters, and delegation or distribution of authority

Contract Research Organization Company that contracts with sponsor to manage some or all aspects of a clinical trial

CRF See case report form

CRO See contract Research Organization

Curriculum vitae A report that outlines the education, work experience, honors, organizational memberships, publications, and presentations of a particular individual

CV See curriculum vitae

Dose-limiting toxicity In a phase I study, an adverse event (usually grade 3 or higher) that is defined as unacceptable and therefore stops further dose escalation

Efficacy An outcome that defines a drug's ability to relieve symptoms or stop the progress of the disease

Evaluable disease   Disease seen on radiographic study that does not have discrete boundaries and therefore is not measurable

Evaluable patient   A patient who has satisfied all protocol requirements and whose outcomes are recorded in relation to the study objectives

Exception   A deviation from the protocol that is sanctioned by the sponsor

Food and Drug Administration   A branch of the Health and Human Services Department of the federal government of the United States, charged with regulating the sale of food, drugs, and cosmetics

GCP   See Good Clinical Practice

Good Clinical Practice   A standard by which clinical trials are designed and conducted to ensure that data is scientifically valid and the rights of patients are protected

Half-life   The time required for a living tissue or organism to eliminate one-half of the substance that has been introduced into it

ICH   See International Conference on Harmonisation

Inclusion criteria   Conditions patients must satisfy in order to participate in a clinical trial

IND   See Investigational new drug

Informed consent   A process in which candidates for clinical trials are given information about the trial and have an opportunity to ask questions; a document explaining all aspects of participation in a clinical trial which is signed by the subject and the person who provided the information as an acknowledgment of receipt of information

Initiation   The process of reviewing all aspects of a protocol prior to enrolling patients

Institutional review board   An institution-specific group of medical and nonmedical professionals who review proposed and existing clinical trials to provide for the safety and rights of research subjects

Intent to treat   A requirement in some protocols to follow patients' survival information for patients who signed the informed consent but did not receive the study drug

Interim analysis   An examination of the data, usually at the midpoint of a study, to review safety and/or efficacy and determine whether the study should continue

International Conference on Harmonisation   A meeting held to define international guidelines for Good Clinical Practice

Intraperitoneal   Within the peritoneal cavity

Intrathecal   Within the spinal canal

Intravenous   Within a vein

Invasion   Extension of cancer cells into surrounding tissues

Investigational new drug   A new drug, antibiotic drug, or biological drug that is used in a clinical investigation

Investigator   The leader of the research team who is responsible for conducting the clinical trial in accordance with Good Clinical Practice and providing for the safety of the study subjects

Investigator's brochure   A proprietary and confidential summary of the preclinical data of a specific study that is supplied to all investigators participating in a clinical trial

Investigators' meeting   A meeting of investigators and study coordinators convened by the sponsor to review a multicentered protocol and related case report forms

IRB   See Institutional review board

Maximum-tolerated dose   The highest dose of a drug that can be safely given to study subjects without unacceptable side effects

Medical monitor   The physician designated by the sponsor who has primary responsibility for the clinical aspects of a protocol

MedWatch report   An FDA-required summary of a serious adverse event which is or may be related to an investigational drug or device

Metabolite   A compound produced by metabolism of the study drug

Metastasis   The transfer of disease from one part or organ of the body to another part or organ that is not physically connected

Micrometastasis   The existence of disease in a part of the body that is not detectable radiographically or by palpation

Monitor   An individual who serves as a liaison between the sponsor and the site by reviewing the progress of the clinical trial by data verification

Performance status   A measure of the patient's functioning in relation to activities of daily living

Pharmacokinetics   Analysis of serum drug levels to define metabolites and half-life

PK   See Pharmacokinetics

Preclinical studies   Testing of the investigational agent in the laboratory and with animals

Presumptive diagnosis   A disease diagnosis made in the absence of clear histologic evidence

Progression   The growth of index lesions by a specified percentage over baseline

Promotion   The second phase in the development of cancer in a cell; the introduction of a carcinogen

Protocol   A written statement of the rationale, objectives, and procedure to conduct a clinical trial

Quality of life   An instrument completed by study subjects to define the patient's daily functioning

Query   An electronically generated question about reported information

Radiation therapy   A treatment for cancer through the use of x-ray or particles from radioactive substances

Randomization   The arbitrary assignment of patients to a specific arm of a study

Refractory   Resistant

Regulatory binder   The official file of a given protocol containing all documents and communication

Restaging   Repeat scanning to determine disease status

SAE   See serious adverse event

Serious adverse event   An event that results in death, a life-threatening adverse event, inpatient hospitalization or prolongation of existing hospitalization, a persistent or significant disability/incapacity, or a congenital abnormality

Shadow chart   A file that contains copies of all pertinent patient information

Site initiation visit   A meeting of study personnel and sponsor personnel that takes place at the site for the purpose of reviewing the protocol, CRFs, study procedures, and the site's facility

Site visit   A visit by the sponsor to facilities that will participate in a specific protocol

Source document   The original document pertaining to a specific patient's treatment

Sponsor   The organization that develops the drug, conducts preclinical research, designs the protocol, and funds the clinical research

Staging   Baseline studies to determine extent of disease

Standard operating procedure   Written statement of policy and/or procedure

Standard treatment   The current therapy generally accepted by the medical establishment for the treatment of a certain disease

Study arm   The treatment determined by random selection

Study coordinator   The person at the site who is responsible for the day-to-day operation of a clinical trial

Study cost grid   A table defining the billing procedures related to a study

Study reference guide   A notebook provided by the sponsor defining study procedures

Subject   A person who volunteers to participate in a clinical trial

Systemic chemotherapy   Drug therapy given orally or intravenously to reach all cells of the body

Tickler file   A chronological file

Toxicity   An adverse effect of a therapy. See Common Toxicity Criteria

Toxicity table   An appendix to the protocol which defines parameters for grading adverse events

Tumor marker   Substance expressed by either a tumor or by normal tissue in response to a tumor; can be found in serum, body fluids, or tissue

Unexpected adverse event   A subject's experience during the course of a clinical trial that was not anticipated

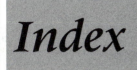

Index